THE WORLD HAS CURVES

THE GLOBAL QUEST FOR THE PERFECT BODY

JULIA SAVACOOL

RODALE

Rodale books may be purchased for business or promotional use or for
special sales. For information, please write to:
Special Markets Department, Rodale Inc., 733 Third Avenue,
New York, NY 10017

Printed in the United States of America
Rodale Inc. makes every effort to use acid-free ♾, recycled paper ♻.

Photo credits: page 26, Honolulu Academy of Arts, Hawaii, USA/Giraudon/The
Bridgeman Art Library. Nationality/copyright status: French/out of copyright;
page 29, Galleria dell' Accademia, Venice, Italy/The Bridgeman Art Library.
Nationality/copyright status: Italian/out of copyright; page 33, Victoria & Albert
Museum, London, United Kingdom/The Bridgeman Art Library. Nationality/
copyright status: British/out of copyright; page 36, Prado, Madrid, Spain/
Giraudon/The Bridgeman Art Library. Nationality/copyright status: Flemish/out
of copyright; page 37, Hermitage, St. Petersburg, Russia/The Bridgeman Art
Library. Nationality/copyright status: Flemish/out of copyright; page 41,
Killerton, Devon, United Kingdom/National Trust Photographic Library/
Andreas von Einsiedel/The Bridgeman Art Library. Nationality/copyright status:
copyright unknown; page 55, AP Photo/Greg Baker; page 60, AP Photo/str; page
101, AP Photo/Collin Reid; page 133, AP Photo/Robert Keith-Reid.
Book design by Christopher Rhoads

Library of Congress Cataloging-in-Publication Data

Savacool, Julia.
The world has curves : the global quest for the perfect body / Julia Savacool.
p.   cm.
Includes bibliographical references and index.
ISBN-13 978–1–60529–938–9 hardcover
ISBN-10 1–60529–938–3 hardcover
1. Feminine beauty (Aesthetics)   2. Beauty, Personal.   I. Title.
HQ1219.S26   2009
306.4'613—dc22   2009023451

Distributed to the trade by Macmillan

2   4   6   8   10   9   7   5   3   1   hardcover

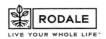

In celebration of the many shapes and sizes

that give the world its curves.

CONTENTS

ACKNOWLEDGMENTS

Writing this book was an adventure of the best sort—one that connected me to the people who daily define and redefine their country's aesthetic particularities and preferences. Along the way, I met many thoughtful women with strong opinions, some with whom I have developed an ongoing friendship. Forming these relationships was also an adventure, as I navigated international time zones, language barriers, and the relative concept of "interview deadlines" in cultures around the globe. I am deeply indebted to all the women who allowed me to experience their world and who opened up their lives and their hearts to discuss a topic as intimate and personal as one's body.

I am grateful for the support of my colleagues, in particular Tara McKelvey for all her advice; Abigail Haworth for her enthusiasm and connections in China and Japan; and Laurie Campbell for her research assistance. Many thanks go to Kate Lee at ICM for believing in this book from the start and finding it a happy home; and to Julie Will at Rodale for her thoughtful edits and eye to detail.

To the various women's and nonprofit organizations that supported this project and helped me forge connections in remote places, thank you. I could not have completed this book without your insider knowledge, especially Women for Afghan Women and Cooperation for Peace and Unity. I would also like to thank Shayma

Daneshjo for being so generous with her time and connecting me with other Afghan women in the United States.

Many thanks to my mother for her ideas and insights. And to Brian Finn, for his tireless encouragement, enthusiasm, and brainstorming sessions (and understanding the many late nights and lost weekends), your support means everything to me.

Introduction

In 2004 I wrote an article for *Marie Claire* magazine titled "Women's Bodies, Then and Now." Based on research and anecdotal evidence, my article was an investigation into the ways in which women's body shapes have changed around the world over the last 200 years. It became one of the most popular features the magazine had ever run, generating letters, e-mails, and stories from readers that reflected the diverse array of ethnicities and heritages that constitute American women. My story had clearly piqued their interest, and perhaps touched a nerve. Finally, a magazine article had asked women to consider their own body size and shape, not based on the expectations of American society, but through the lens of culture, place, and history. The story was intimate and anthropological at the same time: It said, "This is why you look the way you do."

Around the date of the article's publication, *Newsweek* magazine ran a widely noted cover story on "The Global Makeover." In it, the authors profiled one of the world's top models, Saira Mohan, who attributed her commercial success to her decidedly 21st-century pedigree: She's a mix of Punjab Indian, Irish, French, and Canadian.

Mohan is a poster child for the way many Americans think about female beauty. On the surface anyway, we are encouraged to embrace our multicultural heritage, which broadens our definitions of the ideal physical aesthetic. "I think my popularity as a model has to do with the fact that everyone can see a little bit of themselves in me," Mohan said when I spoke with her in my office not long after the *Newsweek* feature was published. "It is not so easy today to say, 'she looks Indian' or 'she looks Italian.' Beauty is truly going global."

But is it really? In recent years, we've seen the globalization of economies, technologies, and politics. Distinctions between cultures are being blurred, so that geographical boundaries no longer determine a population's musical tastes, movie idols, and gastronomic preferences. Sushi in Des Moines? Check. Salsa dancing in Kyoto? You got it. Yet does the same principle apply to women's appearances? Are such standards as easily malleable as trends in automobile styles and hem length? How do different societies define the perfect body?

My research suggests that when it comes to women's body shape and beauty, the world is *not* flat. Our bodies—our most intimate possessions—are also our most obvious means of making a statement. Our bodies speak volumes about individuality and collectiveness, about femininity and feminism, about cultural identity and the acceptance of social standards and practices. The body, to paraphrase Martha Graham, reveals everything. With every gesture, a person is capable of revealing intimate details about self, personality, beliefs, and emotions. Singularly, a person's body speaks to the needs and desires of the individual. Collectively, human bodies help explain the pleasures and priorities of an entire society.

What are women's bodies around the world telling us today? More than anything, they tell us that they are entrenched in the wars of the 21st century: battles over politics, religion, technology, and globalization. In the United States, more than ever, our bodies tell us they are confused. *We* have confused them. We tell them they must be thinner, then overfeed them until they can only grow larger. In 2007, 13 million people in the United States received cosmetic enhancement procedures. More than 400,000 women paid for breast implants. Another 150,000 could be found at one of Jenny Craig's 600 weight loss centers on any given week. And up to 10 million were suffering largely in silence from eating disorders like anorexia and bulimia.[1]

Our drive to achieve "the perfect body" is so pervasive in America that it's become a preoccupation: When you walk past a shop window, you automatically swivel your head to check out your silhouetted reflection. Shopping for clothes, you feel a rush of pride when you can squeeze into a size smaller than you'd expected (a fact of which marketers are well aware; hence the popularity of "vanity sizing"). In America, the ideal body for women is increasingly longer and leaner than seems humanly possible—and, indeed, is frequently not humanly possible, a realization that has given rise to a booming industry of cosmetic procedures, products, and diet and fitness plans. The exception, or perhaps contradiction, to the skinny-is-beautiful trend in America is our fixation on breasts, the only acceptable fat on an otherwise lean body.

The fact that thin is in is an irony not lost on obesity researchers, who report that the average size of Americans has increased 15 percent in the last 10 years. One in five of our children qualifies as obese, and the average weight of an American woman now hovers near 164 pounds (compared to 140 in 1960). To be fair, we're 1 inch taller today as well, standing at 5 feet 4 inches. But even that can't compensate for our ever-expanding waistlines. This reality is comical when juxtaposed with our fantasy body, which is 5 feet 9 inches, 115 pounds, with perky B-cup breasts.[2] Few women look like this to begin with; fewer still come close to the medical definition of ideal weight. Never before has the "perfect" body been at such odds with our true size.

As for who is responsible for creating this American ideal, it's a dicey issue. I would argue *we* are. We—the media, yes, the fashion industry, sure—but "we" primarily meaning you, me, our friends and colleagues, and every American woman of my generation who is actively participating in the creation of an ideal at odds with our reality. We see ourselves as a generation that makes our *own* rules when it comes to using our gender—and our bodies—to our advantage. We believe, thanks to 40 years of feminism that ensured that my generation would be free from others' standards about our appearances, that we can mold and shape ourselves however we choose. That is what our mothers' generation fought for: freedom from a body ideal purportedly created by men, for men. Nearly 20 years ago, Naomi Wolf advocated for an end to this physical double standard in *The Beauty Myth*. And yet, nearly 2 decades later, body image—in America and abroad—needs to be reconsidered in light of a generation of young women who were born with an assumption of equality, who believe we can become CEO or senator or even president.

The pattern I saw in writing this book is that time and again, a woman's body size and shape, in every country around the world, has become the most visible display of financial and social status—her own and her family's. Like designer jeans and luxury cars, the shape of a woman's body in any culture has been commoditized as an immediate indication of class and wealth. This is a global observation: It holds true whether in South Africa, where heavier female shapes are considered ideal,[3] or in Hollywood, where perfection is about molding the human body into an impossible form. Opposite ideals, but in both instances, aspired to by the most affluent and influential sectors of society.

In any culture, the ideal body is a rarefied commodity. It is difficult to achieve, and typically requires money to do so. As my generation of 20- and 30-something American women gains substantial financial power, it has become increasingly possible to purchase a thin, tanned, and toned body; hence, our definition of the perfect body has shifted to an extreme that's still just out of reach. But I don't think—as others have suggested[4]—that women are simply victims of unfair social pressures and standards. I believe that we are complicit in perpetuating these ideas ourselves. We want the social status that a perfect body conveys.

Body as Economic Barometer

In America, the parallel between economic status and body shape preference is fairly direct. But how is this reflected in other cultures around the world? In China, for instance, where the majority of newly minted millionaires are under age 40, extravagant spending on appearance is an important way to indicate where one stands on the financial ladder. The manipulation of the body via plastic surgery is one not-so-subtle indication that you've got cash to blow: Basic operations, such as liposuction, can easily run more than five times the average annual income. In China, as with many cultures, beauty and body aesthetics are interdependent—when I pose the question of what the "ideal woman's body" looks like, I am invariably told about her height and hair texture, body contours, and skin smoothness. As such, I have addressed body and beauty simultaneously at times because in the context of some cultures, it is impossible to extricate the two issues. In the case of China, where a jar of Estée Lauder Future Perfect antiwrinkle cream—the company's most popular product in the Chinese market—costs nearly as much as the average weekly salary, beauty is a mark of wealth. The relative expense of body- and beauty-driven products and services is even more reason for the wealthy to seek them out, as badges of financial success. Which is perhaps why the country with the fastest-growing economy in the world also has the fastest-growing rate of plastic surgery procedures performed on women.

But it's not just beauty products that are going global—though Estée Lauder's success on an international level is just one example of how cosmetic companies have expanded their reach. Other exported American commodities have impacted the conversation about body ideals in unexpected ways. In Jamaica, American goods came early, in the form of a Coca-Cola bottle exported to the small island back in the 1930s. Over the decades since then, the Coca-Cola bottle shape has become representative of female physical perfection in Jamaican culture. ("She's got a Coca-Cola body" is one of the highest compliments a woman can receive.) While the terminology is derived from an American product, the shape it represents is a far cry from our size-zero ideal. In Jamaica, skinny girls are social outcasts. They are mocked, sometimes mercilessly, and have difficulty finding acceptance. The woman with serious curves—who has the dimensions of an old-fashioned glass Coke bottle, and who would be considered overweight by American medical and cultural standards—gets the attention of local men.

In researching this book, I combed through journals, studies, and books to examine the ways that concepts of the ideal body have formed through the lens of economics and globalization. I spoke with economists, anthropologists, sociologists, and psychologists; experts in eating disorders; and purveyors of pop culture. I also talked with dozens of women from multiple generations in cultures as far ranging as Fiji and France, some of whom I have profiled in the book, many others of whom simply served as invaluable insiders, sharing with me a glimpse into their culture's daily habits and less-tangible but equally important ideas about taste, aesthetics, and etiquette. Through their eyes, I came to understand a bit more about the cultures they inhabit and gained a deeper appreciation of the ways in which body ideals have been shaped and have shifted over the past half century.

Global Tour

Over the past 2 centuries in our country, we have seen a reversal of body shape ideals as a symbol of wealth and status: from pale and plump to tan and trim. In Japan, young women are waging war on a conservative society by choosing a new body ideal. The Japanese women I spoke with said that while they mean no disrespect to Americans, their new preference in body shape—bustier and curvier than ever before—doesn't mean that they aspire to look American. What they *really* want, they told me, is not to look like "old Japan."

I also spoke with women from Fiji, where a dramatic shift in body ideals has taken place over the past 15 years. A primary cause for this change can be clearly linked to the introduction of modern technology—specifically, the integration of television into the islanders' homes.[5]

Across the globe in South Africa, women's body ideals are shifting by the day. A fleshy figure is a sign of beauty in some parts of South African society, particularly among women of the upper class. In a country where thinness can indicate illness—especially HIV/AIDS—and where the disease disproportionately affects the poorest populations, women with meat on their bones are the standard of beauty and financial success.[6]

It is impossible to discuss the factors that influence body ideals without accounting for the influence of religion—or more exactly, the politics of religion. How do women whose bodies are obscured by abayas or burkas determine what an "ideal" body should look like? Do they view their figures as objects of beauty and individual expression in the way Western women do? Does the sudden removal of restrictions on displaying one's body in public radically change a woman's notion of beauty? In exploring these questions, I turned to Afghanistan and the recent rise, fall, and resurgence of the Taliban, and with it, women's styles of dress and personal freedoms.

Body and beauty preferences are visible, tangible, and personal ways for each new generation of young women to establish themselves as different from their parents. As with stylistic changes in music and popular vocabulary from one decade to the next, the manipulation of our bodies provides a clear demarcation of what belongs to a generation, whether in Fiji or Florida, downtown Beijing or the heart of the Bronx. Of course, pursuing these ideals takes money, and so, the generational battle becomes a financial one as well.

Ultimately, I turned my eye back to America. What does our fascination with slimness suggest about our cultural values? And what can we learn about ourselves as a society when we are moving further and further away from the image to which we profess to aspire?

Freedom of Choice

With the exception of Afghanistan, every culture explored in this book is one which women's freedoms reign now more than ever. It is precisely *because* of this fact that I find the body shape standards all the more compelling: Given that body ideals are a choice, and that women are free to choose to aspire to them or not, what is driving women's concepts of the perfect body, and how is this idea being informed by the increasing globalization of our world?

There are some very important caveats to this book, or any book of this nature, that I wish to address here. For one, any conversation about something as large and sweeping as body trends and aesthetics requires generalizations. For every woman who fits the stereotypical image for a particular country, there is another who defies it. We know, for instance, that 66 percent of Americans are overweight. That is a medical fact. Not every one of us works in an office where this is true, has a family where this is true, or socializes with a group of friends where this is true. But statistically, it's a sound measurement, and when discussing body ideals and trends in body shapes around the world, I have begun by looking for the statistical evidence of a trend, then built upon that anecdotally and with additional scientific research. Secondly, in many countries, but particularly the developing ones, there is a noticeable difference in attitudes toward body size and shape in cities versus rural areas. In general, the cities are more connected with the ideas and influences of the West; women in the cities tend (though not always) to be more interested in fashion, which comes with a greater predisposition to the "thin is in" mentality. I have sought to look for the body ideal that prevails in a specified culture—in places where the urban life dominates a country's cultural influences, I have looked to the city. In cultures where small-town life still sets the tone, I have focused on rural attitudes. I have not willingly ignored the steady drumbeat of the Western world's encroachment, or the effects of more and more communities around the world swapping ideas online. But I have tried to filter external influences from those that are ever-present, inherent in the fabric of a society.

What Does It All Mean?

When it comes to cultural preferences for body shape and size, the evidence stands against the world being flat. But there *is* a common theme, a flatness, to the way in which the body is used as a social and economic barometer of women's lives. My goal for this book is to offer women a slightly different perspective on a topic that is significantly more intimate than the expansion of corporate balance sheets or the outsourcing of tech services overseas, but nevertheless equally relevant to a conversation about where our world is headed. By looking at national and global shifts in body image and ideals through the lens of economic, social, technological, and political globalization, I think you will agree that today's generation of women has some very encouraging—and also alarming—things to tell us about our future.

For thousands of years, women's bodies have been the subject of admiration, adoration, and subjugation. In this book, they have also become the lens through which we examine cultural identity and global change. What are women's bodies trying to tell us? Let's listen.

CHAPTER 1

How Do We Define *Ideal*?

Beauty, n. *Qualities that give pleasure to the senses or exalt the mind.*

Ideal, n. *A standard of perfection, beauty or excellence.*

—MERRIAM-WEBSTER'S

Before we embark on our global tour, let's start by defining what we mean by "ideal." As with most things pertaining to appearance, the answer is somewhat subjective, and certainly controversial.

Look it up in Webster's, and you'll find that *ideal* is a noun referring to an agreed-upon standard of perfection, often relating to beauty. And beauty, according to Webster's, is a noun that describes the qualities that give pleasure to the senses. Neither of these definitions addresses what these specific qualities are, or who creates the standards by which they are judged. So before we've even begun, already we have a quandary, one that has been mused over and written about for centuries past and centuries to come: When it comes to a woman's body, exactly what constitutes beauty?

Not surprisingly, in the 2,000 years since the birth of Christianity (and for several thousand before that), the answers to these questions have varied dramatically and often contradictorily. Flat, curvy, tall, tiny—all of these characteristics have, at some point, somewhere, been aspired to by a female population. Until the 20th century, cultural opinions and standards related to the female form were largely left to the realm of poets, artists, and philosophers. From Rubens's fleshy, overly ample figures to Gauguin's strong, box-shouldered Tahitian nudes, renderings of the female form were often a matter of the artist's personal preference—or his commentary on society—and left to his aesthetic taste. But in the past 100 years, as science has become the prevailing tool by which our world is explained, the urge to quantify just about everything has spilled over into the realm of beauty. So what has the 20th century revealed about our definitions of ideal? Even now, there is no one perfect answer to the question of perfection. But there are some worthwhile theories. And while I don't believe any one of them holds the answer we are looking for, they are worth exploring, if only to provide some context for our international debate.

It's All about Sex

The first and arguably most popular theory stems from the work of David Buss, PhD, an evolutionary psychologist at the University of Texas who has suggested that our ideas about female attractiveness derive from a Darwinian desire to mate and propagate the species.[1]

According to Buss, "Just as men's successful tactics for attracting women depend on women's desires in a mate, women's attraction tactics depend on men's preferences. Women who succeed in this endeavor appear reproductively valuable by embodying physical and behavioral cues that signify their youth and physical attractiveness. Women who fail to fulfill these qualities lose a competitive edge." In Buss's view, the "ideal" female body conveys to men that she is fertile. In such a Darwinian model, beauty is not in the eye of the beholder; sexual attractiveness is important only insofar as it guarantees that a woman is suitable for reproductive purposes.

As such, a typical "hourglass" figure, with large breasts (an indication of ample food supply for the offspring) and narrow waist with wider hips (a signal of fertility), is ideal. Some psychologists have gone so far as to quantify the ideal waist-to-hip ratio as 0.7 (a waist circumference that is 70 percent of the hip circumference) based on research in which men responded to images of women and ranked them from most to least appealing.[2]

Buss's theory is interesting, albeit highly controversial and somewhat limited. The assumption that men react to specific visual stimuli based on a primal desire to mate eliminates the possibility that women's ideas about their bodies exist irrespective of men's standards. It also suggests that neither women nor men have any conscious influence in the formation of female beauty standards, or that we actively decide what we find aesthetically appealing. Rather, we are at the mercy of a million-year-old evolutionary script.

While this argument may be relevant to regions of the globe in which the need to reproduce is made more immediate by low population density, we are no longer an underpopulated world where one in every five offspring is unlikely to survive. We are an overcrowded population, one that is inflicting irreversible damage on the same natural resources that are necessary to sustain it. Fewer of us, some might say, would improve our planet's odds of survival. If the theory of the evolutionary biologists is correct, wouldn't narrow hips and smaller breasts become hallmarks of the ideal body?

Secondly, under the evolutionary psychology model, body ideals for women are defined as being universal, to the extent that certain physical traits are statistically proven to relate to higher birthrates and better-nourished offspring regardless of ethnicity or culture. So we would expect to see the same body shapes aspired to in Fiji as in Finland. But this is not, in fact, the case. In Japan, as we will see, women used to pad their midsections to create a silhouette akin to a column in order to comply with the preferred look of the moment. In China, women bound their breasts to the chest to create the desired flat look. And in the United States, the obsession with thinness has led to runway models bearing little resemblance to the fleshy ideals put forth by Buss. In a roundabout way, it raises the question: If our body ideals are created to encourage mating, but the obesity epidemic in the United States is driving the female population further and further away from this ideal, why would a society continue to pursue the original ideal? Would it not be advantageous from a reproduction standpoint to alter the ideals so as to encourage men to find heavier women attractive? Taken to the extreme (and, let's face it, evolutionary psychology's theory is extreme), in a world where men only mate with large-breasted, small-waisted, thin-legged women, there won't be much baby-making going on in another

2 decades, because the potential pool of mates is getting smaller and smaller every year.

Further complicating matters, scientists who have studied gender and body image in cross-cultural work have found that the body ideals women aspire to aren't always in sync with the preferred images men choose. The lanky look of Western models is just one example of a body shape that women emulate, though many men prefer the curvier figures on display in *Playboy*. These diverging aesthetic preferences tell us that whatever role evolution may have played in the past, today's ideals are coming from sources other than Darwin.

We Like What's Familiar

Some social psychologists have suggested that we find what is familiar to us to be the most attractive. This theory is based on the assumption that the human brain behaves as a sort of digital camera, photographing and retaining images of every person it encounters. From the day you are born, your brain records and files these images—but not as isolated entities. Rather, each new snapshot is added to the ones before it, then divided by the overall quantity of images, thereby creating a composite of the average woman and man's appearance. The resulting image is the standard by which we judge or perceive the attractiveness of others.[3]

This is more than just an abstract theory: Numerous studies have been conducted in which participants were asked to choose the most attractive faces and bodies from among hundreds of images—some of which were created by computer technology that merged and blended thousands of individual face and body images. Participants consistently selected the composite images as more attractive than any one individual, unaltered photo.[4] As psychologist Nancy Etcoff points out in *Survival of the Prettiest*,[5] "Most people do not conjure up the word 'average' when they see a good-looking face. But average in this context means average in shape, not beauty. In a world of short noses and long noses, almond-shaped eyes and round eyes, oval faces and round faces . . . the eye calculates its own statistics and arrives at a mean value. The beauty of such average may reflect our sensitivity to nature's optimal designs."

It is thought that "average" bodies and faces are optimal because they reassure the viewer that the subject is on solid, healthy ground; overweight people run the risk of heart disease, tall people die sooner, and shortness could indicate malnourishment or a childhood growth stunt. Yet many other physical preferences, from eye shape to breast size to calf muscles, cannot be explained so easily.

Our body aesthetics shift depending on the number of ethnicities with which we come into contact. The American Academy of Facial Plastic and Reconstructive Surgery reports a trend toward preferences for wider noses and fuller lips in the last 50 years.[6] One could argue that these traits have become more prominent in our mental composite as our country's immigrant population swells and the Internet and television introduce thousands of additional non-Caucasian images into our digital memory bank. In their facial composite studies, social psychologists find that Americans increasingly show a preference for features that are less traditionally European. It is tough to discern, though, whether this apparent shift in aesthetic preferences stems from the preference for a true melting pot image, or an appreciation of features that are "different."

But when I spoke with Satoshi Kanazawa, PhD, a psychologist at the London School of Economics and Political Science, he suggested that the criterion people use to choose an "ideal anything" (mate, house, car) is the same: prototypicality. Any item judged to be closer to the prototype is deemed more attractive. In humans, this is the "averageness" effect. I suggested to Kanazawa that the qualities of exceptional height, remarkable thinness, and unusual facial beauty are considered desirable by women precisely because they reflect something *above* average. I asked him if we equate this above-average physical state with other above-average traits, such as higher socioeconomic status.

Yes, he said, for two reasons: "First, taller and more beautiful people are on average more intelligent. They are more likely to achieve higher education and income on their own accord. Second, more beautiful (though not necessarily taller) women are more likely to marry more desirable men who have higher status and more money. So more beautiful women are more likely to attain greater status and more resources via marriage to wealthy men."

Or, without men. Indeed, several studies have borne out the fact that taller women are likely to earn a higher income than women of average height. One study, reported in the *Journal of Applied Psychology*,[7] predicted that workers with a 7-inch height advantage over colleagues would make roughly $166,000 more over the span of a 30-year career. Why? Height leads to greater self-esteem in the individual, while at the same time providing the taller person with a dominating presence in the work environment.

How can it be that we simultaneously find average-looking women the most attractive, while associating certain non-average traits with desirables like money and status? Seeking clarity, I called Jamin Halberstadt, PhD, a social psychologist at the University of Otago in New Zealand, who has received multiple awards for his work on the issue of prototypicality. Halberstadt admitted that the science of averageness is not infallible. He said, "People's judgments do not occur in a vacuum. There is a variability factor depending on what else you have been exposed to in your life. When it comes to bodies, you must account for what the person's own body type is, as well." Perhaps thinner people will prefer thinner people; heavier people will be drawn to rounder shapes. Then again, if someone is dissatisfied with his or her own body type, perhaps he or she sees beauty in someone with the opposite physical makeup.

Emotions also come into play, says Halberstadt. Ask a woman how she feels about her appearance when she's in a good mood, and the response is significantly more likely to be positive (or, at least, less critical) than if you ask her on a day when she's feeling down. The mood–body image correlation is so strong, in fact, that standard medical screenings for depression include questions about how the patient feels about his or her appearance.

If you asked me to describe my ideal body, I would be prone to fantasize. It is not something I possess at the moment, but something I dream about having in the future. An ideal body is about what *could* be, not necessarily what is. To me, this helps explain why, although millions of Americans grow larger every year, our idea of the perfect body continues to shrink. According to the theory of averageness, our concept of the ideal body should reflect the midrange body size in our population; but clearly, if you look at magazines, models, and actresses as evidence of what we find aspirational—it does not.

The Appeal of Being Divisible by Two

Perhaps averageness is not quite the definition of ideal we're looking for. But there's no denying the validity of the many studies that find people are more attracted to composites of faces and bodies than any single image. Researchers from fields as diverse as oral surgery to social psychology sought an answer to why we find these images so appealing, and many of them have arrived at the same conclusion: We are reacting to the science of symmetry. More exactly, the continual blending of individual physical characteristics, over time, will begin to yield a composite that is geometrically symmetrical. Left-eye size evens out with right; people with more pronounced left biceps will pair off with those right-dominant body shapes. Even right and left breast size, which can vary slightly in an individual, become more symmetrical in a composite. Is the ideal body simply perfectly proportioned and balanced?

Twenty-five hundred years ago, sculptors, mathematicians, and philosophers all grappled with the question of how to best capture this principle. What determines proper proportions in human forms, architecture, city planning, and beyond? Plato, Pythagoras, and a myriad of others offered theories, but it was Euclid who appears to have provided the first written description of what became known as the golden ratio: a mathematical formula based on the principles of symmetry that finds the ideal distance between two points and lines intersecting as 1:1.618. Known as *phi* in Greek, the ratio is named after Phidias, an ancient Greek sculptor who designed the Parthenon statues to conform to the golden ratio.

How do we know that the aesthetic ideals employed in building monumental Greek structures 2 millennia ago are the same as those we seek in a human form? Well, we don't exactly. But working backward from the conclusion that symmetry and certain proportions are optimal in our evaluation of beauty, numerous recent studies suggest that there is some truth to *phi*.[8] For instance, an attraction to symmetrical features can be observed in infants, who will stare longer at images of people with symmetrical faces than asymmetrical ones. And research conducted by Randy Thornhill, PhD, a professor of biology at the University of New Mexico in Albuquerque, suggests that adults prefer symmetrical bodies as well, as they associate symmetry in human features with traits such as physical health and strength.

The appeal of symmetry as a tool to gauge attractiveness is that it can be applied to a wide variety of shapes and sizes. A curvy body may have just as much symmetry as a lanky, lean frame; a round face can be just as symmetrical as a square-shaped one, and so on. This may suggest that, despite the fact that different cultures have wildly varying standards of the ideal body, each society's assessment may be rooted in the same criteria.

In fact, a growing number of cosmeticians are making big bucks from the revival of the golden ratio. According to many of them, simple symmetry is only half the story. The rest of it goes like this: The golden ratio creates a series of measured distances, lines that are in perfect relation to one another, whether in the rectangles found in an architectural rendering or in the varying contours found in a sketch of the human face. From antiquity through the Renaissance (it has been debated that Da Vinci employed the golden ratio with the Mona Lisa[9]) to the modern-day research lab of Stephen Marquardt, a California-based plastic surgeon who has become something of the expert in the field of codifying beauty, the lines created by the golden ratio have been used to create a template for physical perfection.

Marquardt's company, Beauty Analysis,[10] uses the ratio of 1:1.618 to create a complex series of lines and angles crisscrossing a frontal grid of the human face that Marquardt calls the Golden Mask. All these lines are symmetrical and maintain the golden ratio—even the ratio between the width of the nose and the width of the mouth is 1:1.618. From his Web site, it is possible to download this Golden Mask and superimpose it on top of a photo of your own face. The places in which your features do not align with the grid (and if you are an average person, there will be many) give you an indication of what a plastic surgeon might be able to alter so that you can come closer to perfect symmetry.

The golden ratio has, as of yet, only been applied to the face. Scientists have yet to draw up a "Golden Cast" for the entire human figure, though individual parts have been assigned the *phi* ratio. In a world obsessed with perfect bodies, though, it's probably only a matter of time.

The World, According to Men

In her now-classic 1991 book, *The Beauty Myth*, Naomi Wolf suggested that female beauty standards aren't determined by biology or math, but have resulted from a full-scale attack on women's position in society. "The beauty myth tells a story," she began in her best-selling book. "The quality called 'beauty' objectively and universally exists. Women must want to embody it and men must want to possess women who embody it. . . . 'Beauty' is a currency system like the gold standard. Like any economy, it is determined by politics, and in the modern age in the West it is the last, best belief system that keeps male dominance intact."

When Wolf's book came out nearly 20 years ago, it was for many women a rallying cry—finally, someone voiced the idea that the pressure to conform to specific beauty standards was a scam, a trap, a way for men to continue to call the shots. Wolf highlighted the correlation between the increased number of women heading to the workplace in the 1960s and '70s and the rise of the cosmetics industry, which, she argues, began to market beauty products to professional women to compensate for the decreasing "housewife market." If women weren't shopping for vacuum cleaners and blenders, what would they buy? According to Wolf, "Somehow, somewhere, someone must have figured out that they will buy more things if they are kept in the self-hating, ever-failing, hungry, and sexually insecure state of being aspiring 'beauties.'"

As Wolf notes, in the years corresponding with the rapid rise of women in the workplace, America launched a $33 billion a year weight loss industry, with another $20 billion being spent by women on antiaging products and self-enhancement services. Wolf concluded that women were being forced to ask themselves whether they wanted to be seen as "sexual or serious"—and that the pressure to choose between the two was intentionally created to keep more women from rising through the professional ranks.

My generation—women who were teenagers when *The Beauty Myth* hit bookstore shelves—grew up with mothers who worked full- or part-time jobs and dads who participated in diaper duty and domestic chores. We'll never know what it felt like to apply to college when the best liberal arts educations were reserved for men. And, for the most part, I think it is safe to say that we do not see our bodies as tools being used against us to undermine our own success. To the contrary, in a world where more and more aspects of everyday life feel out of our grasp and technology is increasingly responsible for how we live and think, our bodies are some of the only things over which we can still exert some control. My generation doesn't view men as the enemy or consider ourselves in any way "less" than those with the XY chromosomes. We enter a conference room with the presumption that we are at least as smart (if not smarter) as the guys sitting across the table. It is not naïveté—we recognize a sexist remark when we hear one and call it out as such when we feel like it. We didn't have to fight the fights of our mothers and grandmothers, most of us are well aware that what they did allowed us to be who we are. We don't buy into the idea that our bodies are the pawns in a giant scheme orchestrated by men to convince us that we are less than perfect.

There's no denying that more women work outside the home now than 10 years ago; more of us are CEOs or other high-ranking executives; more of us are present in government, law, banking, and just about every other powerful profession.[11] And yet you could argue that our fascination with body work and beauty treatments is at an all-time high. One does not seem to stifle the other; rather, they appear to feed off one another. The more successful we become, the more capital we have to invest—and choose to invest—in looking good and feeling good about our bodies.

Like many women of my generation, I am convinced that in a world without men, media, marketing, evolutionary imperatives, or psychological games, we would still pursue the ideal body. What is it, then, that drives us? And how do we formulate our "perfect body" standard? The answer, I believe, is multifold, but is driven significantly by economics and its accompanying social values, including power, status, social hierarchy, and health.

CHAPTER 2

PERFECTION, RECONSIDERED

The natural effort of every individual to better his own condition . . . is so powerful, that it is alone, and without any assistance, not only capable of carrying on the society to wealth and prosperity, but of surmounting a hundred impertinent obstructions with which the folly of human laws too often encumbers its operations.

—ADAM SMITH, *THE WEALTH OF NATIONS,* BOOK IV, CHAPTER V, SECTION IV

Such is the delicacy of man alone, that no object is produced to his liking. He finds that in everything there is need for improvement. . . . The whole industry of human life is employed not in procuring the supply of our three humble necessities, food, clothes and lodging, but in procuring the conveniences of it according to the nicety and delicacy of our tastes.

—ADAM SMITH, *LECTURES ON JUSTICE, POLICY, REVENUE AND ARMS*

Eighteenth-century Scottish economist Adam Smith, a proponent of free-market capitalism and observer of human nature, first explored the idea of self-improvement as an underlying force of economic progress in his groundbreaking book, *The Wealth of Nations,* upon which much modern-day economic theory is based. With the Western world on the cusp of the Industrial Revolution, Smith evaluated the systems in place that allow such progress to happen, and settled on the free-market concept as optimal for economic growth. But *The Wealth of Nations* was more than just an economic treatise—it also explored sociology and psychology. Smith described the basic forces that drive human behavior and explained how the development of highly successful economies is dependent upon a specific set of fundamental characteristics.

In Smith's view, the natural tendency of man is to improve his lot in life; he is born a striver, and his self-interested quest to achieve a certain standard of living—and reach for more—motivates the rest of a society to follow suit. In this way, an individual's pursuits lead to a community of strivers and achievers who come together, not intentionally but organically, as a whole to improve the group's overall standard of living. "The uniform, constant and uninterrupted effort of every man to better his condition . . . is frequently powerful enough to maintain the natural progress of things toward improvement," Smith wrote.[1]

This concept was echoed almost 200 years later in the development of a new branch of psychology during the 1950s. Humanistic psychology, founded by Carl Rogers and others, is rooted in the premise that within every person lies an innate motivation to develop one's potential to the fullest. Rogers referred to this as *self-actualizing*. According to C. George Boeree, a professor of psychology at Shippensburg University in Pennsylvania, who has written extensively about Rogers's historical place in the development of psychology as a discipline,[2] "Rogers captured with this single great need or motive all of the other motives that other theorists talk about." Indeed, Rogers found a way of explaining not only *what* people want to pursue, but *why* they pursue it. Furthermore, he goes on to explore the idea that our quest for self-actualizing is frequently disrupted by influences of a society out of sync with our personal goals, causing us to create an "ideal self"—the person we would likely become if all conditions were optimal. Rogers described the discrepancy between the people we are and our ideal versions as "I am" versus "I should."

Later psychologists have expanded upon Rogers's theory (and some say distorted it), but his premise remains compelling: Left to our own devices, the human tendency is to strive for perfection, or ideal. I think that this concept, proposed by an economist and psychologist alike, is a useful tool to help us understand how various interpretations of the ideal body—in America and abroad—have come to be inextricably linked to the economics of a culture and the social status of women who pursue perfection. It also provides some insight into why our ideals so often seem elusive.

Three Golden Rules

Rarely is a culture's notion of the perfect body in agreement with that population's actual shape or size. In countries ravaged by disease or famine, heavier female figures are generally considered ideal. In a nation that produces 3,900 daily calories for every man, woman, and child, we prize slimness. And almost universally, the preferable body shape increasingly skews toward youthfulness—this as the global life expectancy rises by the year. In the context of bodies, *ideal* has come to mean elite, far-reaching, selective. In basic terms, the body type you want is inevitably the body type you don't have. To that end, I believe that the very definition of an ideal body hinges on three conditions.

First, an ideal body is a shape or size not commonly found among the majority of a population. The ideal figure is noticeably different from the average body size or shape—it exudes a rarefied quality and is considered to be an "improvement" upon the average.

Second, an ideal body does not just happen by accident; it must be a *challenge* to attain. When it comes to body shape, because of the difficulty and rarity of achieving this ideal, those who come close to doing so generally become elevated in social status in their communities. This qualification is important, because it separates the desirable characteristics in an ideal appearance from the merely bizarre. To use an extreme example, consider that not many people in our country have purple hair—it is a rare physical quality. However, if you took a poll, it's unlikely that many people would respond that having purple hair is enviable. One explanation could be that purple hair simply doesn't appeal to our aesthetic sensibilities. But it's also fairly easy for anyone to purchase a cheap bottle of hair dye, spend 20 minutes in the bathroom, and emerge with radically different hair color. A size 2 figure, on the other hand, is neither commonly found in American society nor easily attained. Those who do achieve it are admired for what is interpreted to be a commitment of their resources and a desire for self-improvement. Taken together, the rarity of the ideal and the challenge to achieve it greatly increase its value as a status symbol and as a commodity.

To use a different example, look at how we value cars in our culture, or gemstones. A Porsche or Ferrari looks very little like your average family station wagon and indeed, for every five General Motors cars produced in 2007, less than one Ferrari rolled off the assembly line.[3] Even if every person in America had the means to purchase the sexy Italian sports car, the limited supply ensures that only a select handful will be able to do so. Similarly, a diamond, while sharing a likeness in appearance to a cubic zirconia, is infinitely rarer and more difficult for the average person to purchase due to the higher price. In this context, we can view the ideal female form as a highly desirable commodity, elevated in its allure because of its inherent challenge to obtain. Eager consumers, anxious to make a statement about themselves and their status within a community, pursue it with determination—though only few will be lucky enough to achieve their goals.

And finally, the third defining factor of the ideal body is based on an understanding that those who are able to achieve it must possess an uncommon set of means. Sometimes this reflects internal qualities: drive, ambition, discipline, and willpower. In America, it's clear that this is one reason thin is deified and fat repulsed—more power to the women who can face a dessert tray and wave their hand with a nonchalant "No thanks." We admire these women's control; we admire these women, period. But these idols of self-imposed willpower also garner a good deal of disdain, since their discipline also underscores their dinner partner's lack thereof. "For God's sake, eat some dessert," their girlfriends tell them. "What, are you afraid you'll get fat?" Mocking, taunting, teasing—it's practically a female social ritual for many American women. Admiration and jealousy are frequent bedfellows.

Beyond sheer willpower, achieving an ideal body reflects the possession of a set of external qualities: money, connections, social and political power. Attaining the pinnacle of body beauty is a game for rich girls—or at least, its pursuit becomes significantly easier for those with money to burn. Consider this: The average cost for a tummy tuck in the United States runs between $6,000 and $8,000; liposuction, depending on how much and where, goes for anywhere from $3,000 to $10,000. In major US cities, a health club membership averages between $70 and $85 a month, not to mention the one-time initiation fee, which is often 10 times the monthly rate. Even within the fitness industry, certain memberships are worth more as status symbols than others: The most expensive gyms, like E at Equinox in New York City, cost upward of $23,000 annually (for which you are entitled to perks like personal trainers and towels—heated or chilled—in the locker room). And some club memberships, like those at New York Athletic, can't even be bought—members are selected by invitation only. When you contrast these prices to the average American salary—hovering around $24,000—it's easy to see why the perfect body has become a trademark for women of a certain economic and social class, why many women with decidedly less fabulous lives suggest that they could never look like their thinner, wealthier counterparts. (We say it about celebrities all the time, after all—if only we had their salaries, their personal chefs, their daily one-on-one training sessions, their flexible schedules, we too would undoubtedly look like red carpet material.) And the truth is, no matter what a woman's financial means, body work, over the course of her lifetime, turns out to be one of the most expensive investments she will make.[4] Regardless of nationality, women use their bodies as an indicator of social and financial status, and judge other women by the same standard.

Despite our persistent and aggressive pursuit of the ideal body, however, there is something inherently uncomfortable about acknowledging it. We are more at ease with the concept of commoditizing ideals in other arenas of life (we want the big house, fanciest car, coolest job, sexiest mate), but the thought that we would commoditize ourselves by the same methods leaves us anxious. What is it about the concept of physical perfection that makes women feel so anxious? In *Survival of the Prettiest*, Nancy Etcoff writes, "Envy is hostility toward the very thing one desires. Why is there so much self-denigration and envy? Because every woman somehow finds herself, without her consent, entered into a beauty contest with every other woman." In other words, the hostility some women express toward the concept of the perfect body and those who pursue it might be explained by the fact that, underneath it all, this ideal is something every woman either strives for or believes she's supposed to strive for (or, to use Rogers's and Smith's terminology, "the very thing one desires"). Even if we don't openly admit to seeking the ideal, society positions women in such a way that others would simply assume that she is on the quest. Denial of any interest in pursuing a body prototype saves women, at least on the surface, from expressing anger at their inability to measure up to their competitors and those few women who have already achieved the golden standard.

Meanwhile, the select women who come closest to attaining the ideal body are able to advance themselves in the social and economic pecking order. It creates a conflict for the other women, who may at once admire and loathe those who use their appearances to elevate their status. Admitting envy forces us to own up to the fact that we are playing the game too. It boils down to this: Our bodies are mechanisms by which we express status. And while we're quite comfortable draping them with luxury accessories and designer dresses that not so subtly announce our financial success, we seem to be less open to the idea of commoditizing the body underneath.

In 2001, sociologist Debra Gimlin wrote *Body Work,* a provocative, controversial treatise on what she saw happening in various disciplines of self-improvement, from beauty salons to Spin classes to plastic surgeons' offices. Gimlin's experience was not that women were reluctant participants in these "rituals of body work," as she calls it, nor that they were ambivalent about pursuing their goals. What she did find was an overriding sense of anxiety about other people's perceptions of their desires. "Body work is a double-edged sword," Gimlin explains. "While feeling enormous pressure to look a certain way, [women] also, as feminists, experience tremendous guilt when they respond to these pressures through work on their bodies."[5] That pressure, Gimlin clarifies, is not forced upon women without their consent: "[Body work] has been cited as part of a backlash against women's social and economic accomplishments, interpreted as an attempt (largely male) to enslave them in preoccupation with their bodies and thus limit their capacity even further. I do not share this interpretation."[6] Neither do I. Nor, I think, do most 30-something, college-educated, career-driven women who happen to think a great set of calves would nicely complement their tailored Armani skirt as they hold court at a company board meeting. For this generation, body work is not about giving up one pursuit (career success) in exchange for another. It's about putting icing on our cake (nonfat though it may be)—and knowing we deserve it.

Our Bodies, Our Status

Of course our world remains skewed toward the male population, in everything from salary distribution to medical care. And yes, women are influenced by men's perspectives on attractiveness in potential partners. But women's interest in women's bodies goes hand in hand with their successes in other areas of life. If we can be CEOs and senators and stock investors and single moms by choice, why shouldn't we get the body we want? Why shouldn't we buy the best cosmetics, the nicest clothes, the most expensive haircut? Is it wrong for women to want to surround themselves with the visual cues of their hard work and achievement? If thin, tanned, and toned signals money and status without actually ever saying a word, you bet that today's young and ambitious women will be hitting the gym, pronto.

I asked Gimlin, now a professor of sociology at the University of Aberdeen in Scotland, what it is about the perfect body that we find so irresistible—and why, if we are so seduced by it, few of us come close to achieving it. After all, in the views of Adam Smith, the drive for ideal within each individual ought to uplift society as a whole.

"Slimness in Western culture has become synonymous with youthfulness and class," she tells me. "These are two hugely important concepts in our society that women endlessly pursue." She acknowledges that there are numerous influencers in the creation of body ideals for women, including gender issues and media propaganda. But, she says, women have been able to work within these parameters to turn a negative into a positive. Instead of feeling captive to the gym or the beauty salon, women use the experience of "working on their bodies" to feel good about themselves—it's "me time." "You'll hear women say after a workout, 'I'm taking care of myself,'" she adds. I suspect this is something we'll see more of in the next few years, as the economy sputters and we're forced to reprioritize our spending habits. A new dress that once made us feel attractive and body confident now seems frivolous. But spending money on improving our bodies helps us imagine we're in control of our destiny, stock market be damned.

If the experience of pursuing the perfect body made women feel miserable and downtrodden and defeated before they ever began, the industry would certainly disappear. But instead, health clubs and cosmetics companies provide us with an enjoyable sense of "progress," a feeling that although we may be stuck at size 12, we can still take charge of our bodies and invest in ourselves in a way that makes us proud. This being the case, surely we'll keep buying more of whatever it is that gets us closer to our goal. And we do.

Of course, the beauty industry has a vested interest in keeping the paradox alive between the bodies we have and the bodies we want. One wonders what would happen if all of our bodies were suddenly worthy of appearing on Victoria's Secret catalog pages or the runways of Paris and Milan. What might happen if our reality ever did match our ideal—if, in Rogers's words, our actual and ideal selves met? Would the beauty industry change course and market to yet another body type, in an effort to maintain consumer demand? I doubt it. For sure, the marketer's job is to create a need for its products, but it is hard to imagine an American body ideal that doesn't at least loosely conform to a long and lean shape. Variations may come and go (waifish or curvy, soft or buff), but the bottom line is that for American women, thinness is an indication of more than an aesthetic—it is a statement about their lives.

CHAPTER 3

HOW MUCH IS THIS BODY WORTH?

*Art completes what nature cannot bring
to a finish. The artist gives us knowledge of
nature's unrealized ends.*

—ARISTOTLE

Strolling through the vast corridors of the Metropolitan Museum of Art on a Sunday afternoon, I am greeted by images of human flesh everywhere I turn. The powerful torso of a Greek discus thrower, sculpted in bronze, grabs my eye in the Greek and Roman art wing. Later I come across Rodin's Adam, towering in stature and awesome in strength, in much the same pose. I walk past Degas' dancers and a pastel series of nudes, and down another hallway, I find myself staring up at Rubens's Venus and Adonis—a voluptuous, unclothed Venus who offers passersby a nearly full-frontal view of her abundant rolls of milky-white, dimpled skin. Upstairs I stop and gaze at Paul Gauguin's oils of Tahitian women, painted at the turn of the 20th century when the South Pacific still seemed like an exotic

25

collection of remote islands where life was driven by hedonistic desires, and bare-chested men spent their days chasing girls in hula skirts. And in the modern art section, the naked, coiled body of Patti Smith, photographed in black and white by Robert Mapplethorpe, confronts me with conflicting body language. Is she sullen or seductive? I'm not sure I'm supposed to know.

Nudes may not make up the majority of Western art through the ages, but certainly they create some of the most memorable and lasting images. The human form has been a subject of inspiration for artists since our earliest examples of Western sculpture and

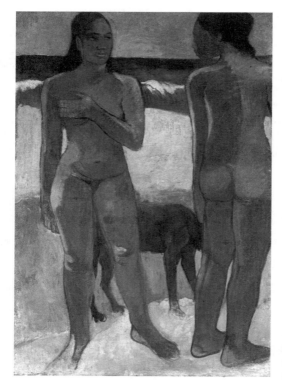

Two Tahitian Women on the Beach, 1891 (oil on canvas) by Paul Gauguin (1848–1903).

painting. In a time before fashion magazines, MTV, and highway billboards, artists' works—on display in private homes and public squares, as adornments to grand-scale architecture and sites of worship—were the predominant means of representing the human body. One can see why the body would be a compelling subject matter: the curves and folds of flesh, the angles and softness, the power of every muscle, and yes, the symmetry of two sides mirroring one another along a center axis. Whether such works were created for commercial sale or civic display, the artist removed the human body from the realm of private conversation and boldly thrust it into the sphere of public opinion.

Looking through the wildly varying representations of the female body throughout the history of Western culture, the question arises: Was the artist's intention to accurately reflect the bodies he observed every day, or to create a physique that he found to be aesthetically appealing, and that may have been distinct from the typical bodies he encountered? In other words, to what extent do time and place influence the artist and his muse? For example, while a photojournalist captures his subject in a dramatic but accurate shot, a fashion photographer may apply his own aesthetic and interpretation to the same subject. As citizens of the 21st century, we recognize this difference in part because we have easy access to television news, the Internet, and fashion magazines and boutiques, which allow us to place the images we encounter in their proper contexts. When it comes to ancient Greek sculptures, we have limited reliable, supplemental images and relatively few descriptive writings on the artists' intent. Instead we have works of marble and bronze, depicting scenes sometimes found in ancient texts and other times illustrating the stories of anonymous men, women, and children that we can only assume are meant to reflect and perhaps comment on the realities of their environment.

When one of these artistic works featuring the human body catches our attention as a particularly beautiful rendering, one wonders if the artist's subject represents an idealized version of physical beauty, his culture's definition of the perfect body, or simply his own artistic vision.

The Greek Influence

It's nearly impossible to examine today's body ideals without taking a closer look at the ancient Greeks. After all, our perception of the body is largely derived from the attitudes set in Athens, 2 millennia ago.

The ancient Greeks quite literally made a science of evaluating the beauty of the human body. The "golden ratio," employed by Phidias in his sculptures for the Parthenon, was a highly popular technique among Greek sculptors. Vitruvius is generally credited with inspiring Phidias's works, and it is the "Vitruvian Man" that Leonardo da Vinci later drew.

During the High Classical period in Greek art, from roughly 480 to 430 BC, artists increasingly began to view the human body as an ideal based on mathematical formulas that could determine proportional perfection. A prime example of this ideal, heavily reliant on the concepts of symmetry and anatomical accuracy, is frequently cited in the creations of the sculptor Polyclitus of Argos. Polyclitus's most famous work, *Doryphoros*, shows a young soldier bearing a

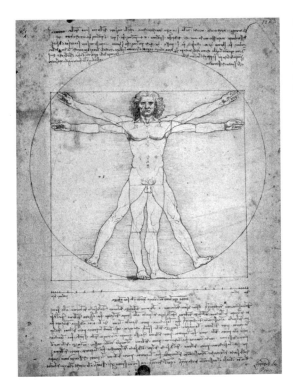

The Proportions of the Human Figure (after Vitruvius), c. 1492 (pen and ink on paper) by Leonardo da Vinci (1452–1519).

spear. The broad shoulders, chiseled abs, and strong, muscular limbs embody not only the anatomical idealization of a male body, but also the narrative of a heroic young warrior heading into battle (some have also interpreted it as an athlete preparing for competition). The Greek portrayal of the human body, rooted in the Platonic belief that for all things there exists an *ideal form*, provides a basis for much of our modern-day ideas about physical perfection.

"What you see in ancient Greece is an effort to glorify the human form in much the same way that the subject matter himself has been glorified for his heroic feats," says Andrew Szegedy-Maszak, PhD, a professor of classics at Wesleyan University in Middletown, Connecticut. "It is clear the Greeks were preoccupied with the concept of beauty—they considered it a treasure," says Szegedy-Maszak. "You'll see endless Greek vases with the image of a young boy painted on [them], and next to him the words '*kalas*' or 'beautiful.'"

Hold everything. Young boy? Where are the sexy women? The quick answer: almost nowhere to be found in the art of antiquity, at least in the realm of nudes and body-focused works. From sculptures to vase paintings to remnants of classical texts, the discussion of bodily perfection focuses on male beauty. Women's bodies were considered weak, infirm, and, in short, not worthy of idealizing. Thus, the vast majority of information we have today about the physical realities and aesthetics of the Greeks pertains to men, not women.

After all, these men spent hours at the gymnasium, competing with other men in various sports and participating in very early forms of strength training. All this was done, incidentally, in the nude (save a small sack worn around the waist) and while heavily oiled. Vain? Maybe, maybe not. For Greeks, the body symbolized more than just one's self. According to Simon Goldhill, a professor of Greek literature and culture at the University of Cambridge, philosophers such as Socrates viewed the upkeep of one's body, in part, as nothing short of an obligation to the entire community—a requisite part of civic pride. "There is no activity in which you will do worse by having a better body," Socrates once said. A person's goal, therefore, should be "to see how you can develop the maximum beauty and strength for your body."[1]

This pride that the Greeks invested in their physical condition—and that we see in their depiction of bodies—can be partially attributed to their devotion to public life. In this cradle of democracy, it was imperative that every Greek appeared "willing to serve"—whether in government, the military, or in weekly sporting contests held in public venues. Did an artist's bronzed gods create the same body image tensions for the everyday Athenian as swimwear billboards or Victoria's Secret catalogs do for us? We have no evidence one way or the other, really. But Szegedy-Maszak points out that the Greeks were an incredibly competitive culture, which is apparent everywhere from the myth of Achilles and Odysseus to the creation of the Olympic games and the courts of law. There were great prizes to be won by the victors of any athletic competition, including an improvement in social status. Furthermore, the Greeks viewed their gods as "completely anthropomorphic," says Szegedy-Maszak. "From the Greeks' perspective, the only difference between themselves and their gods was that they died and their gods didn't." Were there an Athenian version of *Us Weekly*, its popular column might have read "Gods: They're Just like Us," for all the very human mistakes and blunders Greek gods were known to have committed. In other words, though they were literally put on a pedestal, it's possible that in the artwork depicting the awesome muscular power of Zeus or Aries, the Greeks saw a body that was not so impossible to attain and an ideal that encouraged their competitive instinct.

And even in democratic Greece, the human body was far from immune to the influences of class and money. Though it's true that many public arenas were adorned with sculptures of athletes and mythological heroes, so too were the private homes of the elite. To be immortalized in a statue that reflected the symmetry of your body and the beauty of its proportions was an ultimate status symbol. And the only way someone outside the upper class might have a chance to be chiseled into marble was through significant athletic achievement—success in this realm meant he would become a de facto member of the elite. Under these circumstances, the idealized body would have to be one strong enough and fit enough to succeed at whatever physical competition was required.

Barring such athletic prowess, if you were a member of the social elite, it's likely that you were a collector of such works, not a subject. Decorating a home with sculptures of young male beauty allowed its owner to display his aesthetic taste (no small matter to the Greeks) as well as his wealth and his connections. They also served as ancient versions of bodybuilding posters, providing him with a tangible example of what he might one day achieve, with enough time spent at the gymnasium.

The Influence of Fashion

From male muscle to female curves—when did the fascination with the perfect body become focused on women? The answer is not completely clear, but one factor most historians do point to is a dramatic shift in style of dress beginning in the mid-14th century. During the Middle Ages, men and women in much of Europe wore similarly fashioned garments: long, loose-fitting robes that varied in size but not cut. They were, for all purposes, unisex. In the 14th century, that style began to change noticeably. Men began to wear a shorter jacket that

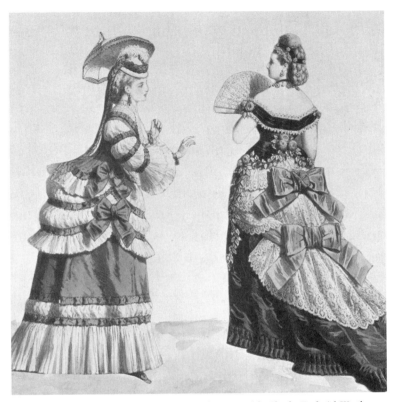

Fashion designs for women from the 1860s (colored engraving) by Charles Frederick Worth (1825–95).

connected with leg-skimming breeches. Women's garb, while still long in length, became much more tailored to the body; the neckline took a serious dip. The result was a new emphasis on the breasts and hips. Though the origins of this shift in design remain unclear, the fact is that it was an instant hit in western and northern Europe, spreading from one territory to another with remarkable speed in the middle of the century. It would be another 600 years before fashion once again toyed with the idea of androgynizing the dress code.

But gender-specific dress was just the beginning of fashion's influential role on body shapes and definitions of ideal. As social philosopher Gilles Lipovetsky notes in *The Empire of Fashion*, "[Fashion] has unleashed an investment of self, an unprecedented aesthetic self-observation. Fashion goes hand-in-hand with the pleasure of seeing, but also with the pleasure of being seen, of exhibiting oneself to the gaze of others." The increasing social value on being "fashionable" played right into our narcissistic tendencies, he believes, allowing us to spend more time focusing on how we looked wearing clothes, and without them. Fashion, like the body itself, speaks loudly to the casual observer about who a person is, what class she belongs to, and how much money she has at her disposal.

Lipovetsky points out that women are generally more concerned with detail than men, and as such are particularly eager consumers of fashion. We discuss the thighs we love, but the love handles we hate; breasts we wish were bigger and bottoms we'd prefer were smaller. I can even recall a conversation with a friend who felt her ring finger was a tad stubby. We are equally particular about our clothes, which ostensibly accentuate or veil each body part we love or hate. We like the neckline, but wish the skirt fell just a bit lower; adore a pair of pants that fit snugly around the hips, but wait—are they *too* snug? Just snug enough? Is there another mirror in the store where we can assess the snugness? Fashion becomes yet another means by which our bodies are assessed. As art historian Kenneth Clark points out in *The Nude*, "Every time we criticize a figure, saying that a neck is too long, hips are too wide or breasts are too small, we are admitting, in quite concrete terms, the existence of ideal beauty."[2] Fortunately for those of us in pursuit of *phi,* fashion can compensate for our self-scrutiny, offering us clothing designed to mask any perceived body flaw.

Women Get Naked

While innovations in 14th-century European fashion may have precipitated the gradual shift in focus from the male to the female body, they are mirrored by a transition in art from male to female nudes. Part of the shift in gender interest, Clark suggests, may come from a decline in emphasis on the study of anatomy in an artist's training, and a rise in focus on the "sensuous perception of [the body's] totalities." Clark offers another explanation that bears considering: the simple fact that women's bodies are more interesting for an artist to contemplate. Where the idealized male nude is full of straight lines and right angles, women's figures curve from one region to the next, making an artist's composition "more harmonious."[3]

Such curvy lines of the female physique perhaps required less rigidity in the geometrical perfection of the body shape on the artist's part, and slowly the emphasis changed. By the 16th century, a style known as naturalism openly dismissed mathematical models of human proportion and principles of symmetry in favor of portraits that appeared to distort the female body in provocative ways. (As Sir Francis Bacon remarked during this time, "There is no beauty that hath not some strangeness in the proportion.") The naturalists' 17th-century successors, the mannerists, would later suggest that beauty stems from the deliberate emphasis of a body part thought to be especially tantalizing.

Not everyone was comfortable with this aesthetic, and in

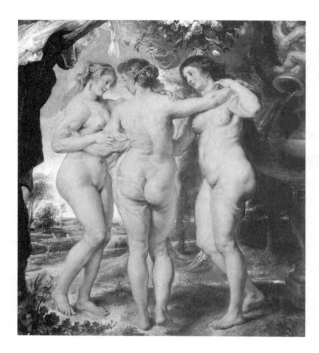

The Three Graces, c. 1636–39 (oil on canvas) by Peter Paul Rubens (1577–1640).

particular, its sexual implications. When Flemish painter Peter Paul Rubens first introduced his visions of women's bodies through a series of nudes, the word "vulgar" was often provoked. Rubens was as riveted by the bulges, wrinkles, and dimples in a woman's skin as he was by her slender neck or ankles. His portraits of ample flesh evoke a strong sensuality.

In his *Three Graces,* the women are decidedly feminine, playful, and angelic; they are also saggy and dimpled and potbellied. In his *Perseus and Andromeda,* the damsel in distress is hardly ideal by our standards today: She has arm jiggle, saddlebags, and cellulite. Was Rubens's intention to display his personal aesthetic, or to comment in some way on the women of the time? Clark suggests that Rubens

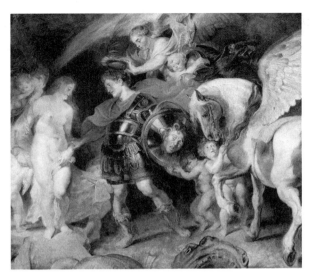

Perseus Liberating Andromeda, c. 1620 (oil on canvas) by Peter Paul Rubens (1577–1640).

painted his women a larger size because it would create a more dramatic moment for the viewer. "Even if he had not felt a natural fondness for fat girls," Clark writes, "he would have looked for accidents of the flesh as necessary to his system of modeling."

These Curves Have Status

By the 19th and 20th centuries, the influence of economics in visual art becomes more obvious. Just as the impressive physiques of young Greek athletes carved into marble served as a reflection of the subjects' elite social positions, the robust female figures of 19th-century portrait paintings were also intended to convey family power and wealth.

In these paintings, many of which adorned the homes of European nobility, the well-padded figures of the ladies of the house—the wives of wealthy industrialists and banking barons—have not been trimmed down by the artist. Unlike the Romans and Greeks, who were sometimes known to sculpt a new head for their subject and place it atop a previously chiseled body, the 19th-century artist paints his well-heeled, well-fed female subject as she is, presumably because she has no reason to be displeased with the accurate representation of her figure.

From 1750 to 1850 in Europe, the Industrial Revolution was in full swing. While only 17 percent of the European population lived in cities in 1801, by 1851, the percentage had increased to 35 percent, and by 1891, it had swollen to 54 percent. Infrastructure and social services simply could not keep up with the influx of new city dwellers. In metropolises like London and Paris, disease ran rampant, the lower class lived in squalor, and famine lurked behind every corner. The general lack of sanitation, accumulation of sewage, and high rates of crime made city living a gritty choice for the labor class. Heavy use of coal meant the air was constantly filled with dirt and grime. In such a society, revolution by the masses was always a threat. In an age when photography was only just being invented (and even then, limited in availability), artist-rendered illustrations were used in newspapers, which were distributed for free or a few cents on busy street corners. These artistic renderings not only added beauty to the page, they also provided social observation and commentary. The body became a tool by which artists could capture and narrate the strife of the urban poor. And what they captured was this: Short of nutritious food and healthy living environments, women of the labor class were waiflike in appearance. Such a body type was indicative of manual labor, be it in factories or farms, under the hot sun or in front of coal furnaces. And given such conditions, the body of the laborer was also rightly depicted as susceptible to the numerous diseases that plagued Europe throughout the century.

Of course, it's not implausible that thinness could simultaneously be a byproduct of an impoverished life, but also be considered attractive. Refuting this notion, however, is an interesting study conducted by psychologist Viren Swami, PhD, at the University of Liverpool in England. Entitled "The Influence of Resource Availability on Preferences for Human Body Weight and Non-Human Objects," the researchers set about measuring how attractive men found different female body types, correlating the data to the participant's hunger level.[4] They found that the hungrier a person was, the more desirable they found heavier women. Swami speculates that this correlation indicates a preference for fuller figures during times of poverty and food scarcity, and conversely, the preference for a thinner female figure tends to coincide with times of economic boom.

In a 2002 paper in the *British Medical Journal* entitled "Poverty and Painting: Representations in 19th Century Europe," authors Philippa Howden-Chapman, an associate professor at the Wellington School of Medicine and Health Sciences at the University of Otago in New Zealand, and Johan Mackenbach, a professor at the University Medical Center in Rotterdam, Netherlands, debate the significance of socially oriented art in the 19th century that used the human body to convey the plight of the average person.[5] They point to works that reflect the physical effects of epidemic diseases such as tuberculosis and syphilis, such as Joaquin Sorolla y Bastida's disfigured faces in *Sad Inheritance*, or Christian Krohg's gaunt-looking character in *Sick Girl*. Gustave Courbet's *Funeral at Ornans* is notable for its "unsentimental focus on the pervasive reality of early death." The social unrest in many countries during this time played out on the political front, and the fall of the Paris Commune led to several paintings of the heroic resistance put up by the workers, 30,000 of whom were killed. In these series of paintings, the female body is depicted as undernourished, wan, and fragile. As the researchers note, "The images show the tensions inherent in varying responses to the poor and their health problems—religious charity, humanistic civility and reform, or revolutionary identification. The representations of poverty in 19th-century paintings show how poor housing, bad working conditions, and chronic hunger cause ill health and early death, showing that artists clearly saw the fundamental causes of ill health and brought them to wider public attention."

If this is how illness and poverty are portrayed, how does the artist convey wealth and prosperity on his canvas? Ingres frequently portrayed his female subjects as amply full-figured, whether an actual portrait of nobility (*The Countess of Touron*) or anonymous women assuming an idealized version of femininity (*The Source* and *The Bather of Valpincon*). The shade of skin color was equally indicative of status, with women of the upper class displaying porcelain skin, untouched by the sun. Even though more women of the labor class were spending their days toiling in a factory instead of in the fields, it was hard to break the association between back-breaking agricultural work in the fields and the leathered, darkened skin tone of the European laborer.

When it came to the development of an aesthetic ideal, as Europe did, so did America. The 19th century on this side of the pond was tumultuous, as the country's fledgling democracy faced the Civil War, the Gold Rush, and increasingly industrialized cities. The Vic-

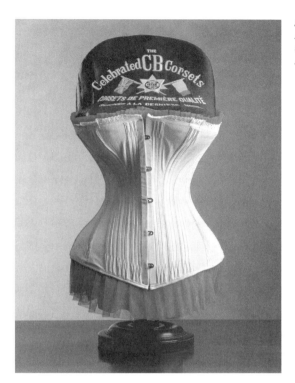

Shop display corset with slogan, "The Celebrated CB Corsets," 19th century (photo).

torian era, so-called because of England's queen, was notable in the United States for its influence on fashion and body preferences. Though its social customs were often perceived as prudish, the Victorian lifestyle was not exactly sexually conservative. The introduction of the corset and bustle in women's clothing ensured that the female body could now be squeezed and plumped to emphasize her most sexual body parts.

Up to this point in Western culture, women's bodies had not been forcefully manipulated to assume an unnatural form or size (though in other cultures, as we will see, the deliberate alteration of body shape has a long history). The corset and bustle said two things to women: Your natural shape is not fashionable; and with a little investment, you can get the body you want.

Today's Ideal

Kate Moss. Paris Hilton. Gisele. The women who make beaucoup bucks showing off their bodies these days share certain necessities: They're tan, toned, and tiny (width-wise, anyway). The pinnacle of body beauty in America can be observed everywhere from runways to advertisements to the chic women in skimpy outfits gathered outside Manhattan nightclubs. Those size-2 figures, the envy of every average-size woman in America, say "almost perfect."

Far from the squalor and poverty that faced the citizens of a nation experiencing the growing pains of industrialization a century ago, America emerged from two world wars richer, stronger, and more economically optimistic than ever. Resources once available only to the elite—restaurants, clothing boutiques, hair salons— became affordable to the masses. Today we are a country with a limitless quantity of cheap sustenance (just witness the 99-cent menus at Burger King and McDonald's). The average job in America for the working class does not involve tilling the fields or standing for 14 hours a day in a factory assembly line. Instead, we sit—at office desks, tollbooths, customer service centers—and expend relatively little energy as we go about our jobs. We spend 40 hours a week under fluorescent lights, staring at computer screens and counting down the hours until dinnertime. Our appetites have grown along with the availability of cheap food, but our ability to burn off the extra energy consumed has not.

In a culture of drive-everywhere, work-inside, shop-inside, eat-inside, there is nothing rarefied about white skin and a robust middle section. After all, two out of three of us are sporting something rather like this look right now.[6] Pale and pudgy have become symbols of America's working class. But this time, there is an additional twist: We don't *have* to have this body type, in the way that a 19th-century factory worker or farmer was bound to be thin and tanned. We could eat less; we could exercise more, even those of us working night shifts and long-hour desk jobs. Because of this, in addition to an overweight body being a symbol of the working class, it has also become associated with something far more stigmatizing: laziness.

In a recent study in the *Personality and Social Psychology Bulletin,* scientists measured the cultural attitudes toward fat people in six countries and compared this to the population's actual body size. They found that while the United States ranked second highest in body mass index (BMI) numbers, it also ranked second highest in the belief that fatness was not a culturally acceptable aesthetic and highest in people's personal fears of becoming fat themselves. The reasons cited ranged from fatness being equated with laziness or lack of intelligence to the perception that overweight people simply "didn't care" about living a healthy lifestyle. According to the researchers, "A significant portion of [fat] prejudice is based on . . . holding group members responsible for negative stereotypic behavior." (The study cites similar examples of stereotyping Hispanic Americans as lazy and Southerners as bigots.) In this way, size in America has become the proverbial double-edged sword. Not only are you assumed to be less financially successful if you have a bigger shape, you are also presumed to be something of a slob—unwilling (not unable) to do something about your appearance.

Tanning requires a concerted effort, an investment of time that the working class does not have. A bronzed glow sends the message "I have time to bathe under the sun, and the money to travel to a tropical destination. I am a member of the leisure class." What 200 years ago was a sign of working in the fields is today a sign of lounging in them—literally—engaged in the leisurely pursuit of "tanning."

Of course, creating this ideal and living up to it are not the same thing, and in many ways the ideal we have chosen for ourselves is becoming increasingly elusive for the average American woman. But rather than give up the chase, we've buckled down and become more fixated than ever on reaching that golden standard. Our desire for the perfect body, from the beginning of Western culture up until the 21st century, cannot be underestimated. Only this time, we're losing ground on the very images we've created for ourselves.

CHAPTER 4

SHOW ME THE MONEY

Personal beauty is a greater letter of recommendation
than any letter of reference.

—ARISTOTLE

Jogging along the East River in lower Manhattan during the early morning hours, I am greeted by a familiar sight: dozens of middle-aged and elderly Chinese immigrants who have emerged from their apartments and walked to the island's edge. They face east, into the sunrise, and acknowledge the dawn of a new day as they perform a series of tai chi moves strung together in slow, fluid, hypnotic motions. Many of them are dressed in traditional Chinese garb—their neutral-toned, loose-fitting blouses and matching shin-length pants rippling in the morning breeze. Together, their lithe, narrow frames expand as they stretch side to side and top to bottom. Not a single one, in the countless times I've observed them as I run by, looks overweight.

A few blocks later, I come across a group of 60-something-year-old women, venturing from the nearby senior center for their morning dose of calisthenics. Wearing sweatpants, tennis shoes, and oversize T-shirts, they look every bit the American grandmother stereotype, right down to their short, permed curly white hair and their padded midsections. As they bend over to touch their toes (which none of them can actually reach), they are jolly looking for sure; ethereal, they are not.

I find the contrast between these two groups always striking. Of course it is anecdotal evidence at best, and I'm aware that the tai chi practitioners are made up of a small sampling of Chinese Americans who still have close ties to the customs and habits of their homeland. It's also true that many of them live near or below the poverty line in New York City, and the glut of fancy restaurants the city has to offer is far from their reach. But still it intrigues me that these hardworking immigrants, many of whom have physically demanding jobs with hours that stretch well past the traditional 9-to-5 office day, rise before the sun to exercise. Their sense of discipline is not one that, frankly, most Americans possess.

Chinese women are no strangers to cultivating willpower, whether for predawn rituals or to withstand their cultural trends in beauty (foot binding is just one example). But until very recently, slimness for women in this Communist country was as much a matter of circumstance as an active pursuit. I spoke with a Chinese woman in her late forties who said simply, "We were all given the exact same amount to eat, day in and day out. And it was never enough. So what do you expect? It is no wonder we all shared the same thin bodies."

In the context of Chinese history, the influence of Chairman Mao's rule is relatively tiny—China, after all, has one of the longest continuous narratives of any country in the world, dating back as far as 5,000 BC. It is a history marked by violent power struggles and political upheavals from one dynasty to the next; and with each change in leadership came a strict set of rules governing dress, behavior, and language. Perhaps because so many different ethnic groups have come to be assimilated under one name (currently 10 different languages are recognized in China and 43 official dialects of Chinese are spoken, though local variations push that number over 100), these shifts in power were dramatic.

When Mao Zedong stepped into power in 1949 and the country was renamed from the Republic of China to the People's Republic, the hardships inflicted upon the average citizen were extreme. During the height of the Cultural Revolution, any method of personal grooming was considered counterrevolutionary, and therefore illegal. Women who owned hairbrushes or makeup, or who were caught painting their toenails, were beaten or forced to endure other methods of public humiliation. Such behavior was considered "bourgeois" by the government—code for "people with money who think they are above the goals of the common society." In compliance with the new look of Communism, women cut their hair short and dressed in identical, drab-colored shirts and pants, known as Mao suits. Any sort of vanity product, from lipstick to body creams, was discarded. "My mother told me how she used to apply pork fat to her face in the winter to keep her skin from drying out because it was against government policy to own lotion," says 22-year-old Niu Mu. Those who did not comply with the look or mind-set of Communism were rounded up and sent off to "reeducation camps";

those lucky enough to eventually return were psychologically trau-
matized from the experience and often incapable of ever finding
their footing in their families or communities again. No one wanted
to stand out from the group—individuality, even inadvertent, could
spell trouble.

A Comrade's Body Ideal

Brute force was one way Communist leaders established a new
code of living, but based on their tumultuous history, I'd argue that
the Chinese people themselves had already learned to adapt to the
harsh daily impacts of new leadership. When the Manchu seized
power in the 17th century, they forced men to grow queues for their
hair—a look that required shaving hair high up on the back of the
head and growing remaining locks into a long, braided ponytail.
Those who refused were executed. And as far back as the 10th century, emperor Li Yu ordered his mistress to bind her feet (ostensibly
so that she would remain "bound" to his side), triggering a painful
practice that lasted more than 900 years. Over the years, tiny feet
eventually became symbols of beauty.

And yet, when it came to ideal body shape, little changed among
Chinese preferences until this past century. "Historically, the preference was for slim women with rounded bellies," says Susan Brownell,
PhD, an anthropologist at the University of Missouri at St. Louis. In
fact, the Chinese coined a term for this shape—*feng man* or a "modest touch of fullness"—to describe a woman's midsection. Such a figure was seen as representative of a woman's *qi* or vital energy,
believed to have its central reservoir in the abdomen. "This rounded
shape was considered attractive because it was associated with

a woman's sexual desire, fertility, and strength," says Brownell.[1]

Fast-forward to 2009. Rounded stomachs? Please. Billboards lining the crowded streets of Beijing and Shanghai advertise one of the fastest-growing industries in the country: cosmetic surgery. And at most clinics, one of the top-five most-requested procedures is abdominal liposuction. How did the ideal woman's body get from there to here?

In a word: Communism. "During the Cultural Revolution in the 1960s, you started to see the backlash against this more feminine figure," Brownell tells me. "Softness and roundness, as physical attributes, were discouraged. An angular, masculine body ideal was favored because it was associated with revolutionary fervor; women emulated the male model because such an appearance was also associated with hard work and manual labor, two things the Communist Party stressed."

Of course, living conditions also necessitated the lean body that had become ideal. As one middle-aged woman told me, "My sister and I used to catch cicadas from the hillside to eat—we had nothing." Unlike other countries, such as South Africa, where a lack of sustenance has encouraged the idealization of a fuller figure, in China, the softer look of previous generations rapidly became unpopular. Political ideology played out in physical ideals, and body types came to reflect the idealized lives of the worker, a trend that persisted for 3 decades until the government began easing trade policies in the 1980s. I talked with many women who grew up during the waning years of Communism's rigid dress-code policies about how their experiences shaped their ideals about body and beauty.

Lijia's Story

*My grandmother used to bind her breasts flat
to her chest. Now young women are getting cosmetic
surgery to make them bigger.*

—LIJIA ZHANG, 44, WRITER, BEIJING

I grew up on the edge of Communism. My mother was a factory worker, and I dropped out of school so I could inherit her job at the age of 16. But as I came of age, you could already see the old Communist rules were changing.

During Communism, any expression of individuality or social class was banned. Foot binding, for years popular among concubines and other types of "kept" women, was outlawed after 1949. I still remember my grandmother's feet—so tiny, as she had practiced the tradition when she was younger and she was a prostitute. Foot binding is a classic example of the Chinese mentality—women are willing to become literally incapable of walking for the sake of appearing a certain way.

By the 1980s, when I was a teenager, China began to go through major reforms. Everything was changing, especially in a woman's ability to express her individuality, so long as she did not say anything critical about the government. This translated into more modern clothing and brighter colors, quite a contrast from the Iron Maid model we had under Mao, where girls all wore their hair in pigtails and dressed in gray, shapeless uniforms.

When I was growing up, physical assimilation was so

strongly encouraged that any little difference in our appearance was scrutinized for deeper meaning. I have always had naturally wavy hair, but that is not common in China. So my boss at the factory thought I had gotten a perm—which was interpreted to indicate my desire to be bourgeois and elitist. Everything had a political undertone to it back then.

My older sister once told me, "The bird who flies first gets shot first." She was always trying to warn me not to work so hard at being different from everyone else. It was safer to blend in. But that's not who I was. I owned a leopard print jacket that I wore sometimes, even though I knew the people at the factory wouldn't like it. But change was coming to China, and it happened on a superficial level first—so long as you didn't criticize the ideology of the Party, you were allowed to show glimpses of individuality.

The traditional image used in China to describe a beautiful female body is that of a weeping willow tree: long and graceful. Women should be tall, but not taller than men. (It's funny; in the personal ads in China, men always include two things: the exact amount of money they make and their height.)

Beyond these body requirements, a woman's ideal appearance in China is as much about her face as it is her body. Double eyelids have always been desirable, as have big eyes and fair skin. Contrary to what people think, the preference for pale skin is not because women want to look Caucasian; rather, it comes from centuries upon centuries of class distinction between the poor people who work in the field and have darker skin due to sun exposure and the wealthy families who can keep their skin lighter. Also, the color of your skin is an indication of your ethnic group and therefore social standing. My skin tone has never been light.

Once, growing up, a relative asked me, "How come your sister is so beautiful, and you are so ugly?" Another time, my father commented that they must have pulled me off a coal pile because my skin was so dark.

It is amazing to see how much has changed in Chinese women's approach to beauty in the last 20 years. Now there are plastic surgery places everywhere in the cities. For a fee, women can get higher nose bridges, bigger breasts, or rounder eyes. Another popular trend is "bone breaking," where women will have their leg bones shattered and a metal rod inserted, in order to gain a few inches in stature. Height is considered a sign of economic power. It reminds me of foot binding: the pain we will endure for the sake of vanity. Everything you need to look "perfect" is available for a price—women are not ashamed or secretive about getting cosmetic surgery, because doing so is an indication of wealth.

Women are increasingly getting breast implants—it's the new look women want. And when I think that my grandmother used to tie cloth strips across her chest to bind her breasts flatter . . .

Overall I'd say women have become much more assertive in what they want, as far as their bodies are concerned. They want the right to express their individuality, and appearance is one way to do that. My generation still knows *the shadow of Communism. For young women in China now, they are free from the fear.*

Communist Backlash

Two hundred years ago, it was possible for a country to close itself off from any meaningful contact with its neighbors, and to shield its people from falling prey to "harmful" external influences. Slow forms of communication, limited travel, major language barriers: All of these worked to the advantage of governments trying to maintain control of their often-restless populace. Images of unruly Americans or dignified Europeans were perpetuated not through firsthand knowledge so much as hearsay and rumors. But the arrival of 20th-century innovations, including radio, planes, trains, and automobiles—and later television and the Internet—blurred time zones, geographical divides, and language barriers. Cultural isolation (North Korea notwithstanding) was fast becoming impossible—not necessarily because governments wanted to be more open, but because the people now had technology on their side.

For China, this meant that while women continued to hide their hairbrushes and don peasant scarves as they conformed to the status quo, they were aware of the world beyond their borders. Government propaganda washed over the airwaves, but so did underground chatter about Western democracy and the great wealth found in nations such as the United States. While famine swept through China's countryside, images of the opulent lifestyles of America's rich and famous—think Marilyn Monroe, Jackie Kennedy—could be found if you knew where to look in Beijing. It's hard not to salivate over the good life you've never had, but it's even harder to resist the pull of a life you used to know; and for many Chinese citizens during the Mao years, memories of their families' happy middle-class lifestyle pre-Communism were all too recent.

And so the Chinese consumer was primed when, in the 1980s, the government began to show signs of relaxing Maoist regulations. *Kaifong zhengce* or "open policy" was the government's mandate to accelerate economic development through importing Western business. Slowly, established American brands such as Levi's and McDonald's began testing China's retail waters. But could the American beauty business succeed in a country where women had for decades been trained to dismiss the concept of self-enhancement? And would Chinese women welcome beauty advice from a foreign adversary? With a healthy dose of wariness, some of America's biggest names in cosmetics invested product research and development funds in China. The challenge soon became evident: Here was a population with a fundamental lack of appreciation for the "science" behind beauty— the very thing that convinces American consumers that a product is worth purchasing. Most women in China were still creating facial concoctions straight from their own kitchens, mixing dyes from various plants to achieve a rosy color for the cheeks or combining oils to moisturize their skin. Anti-retinols and SPFs were of little interest.

So Western companies got creative. The selling point was not in the cutting-edge technology that made their serum the "best" for women, they realized, but in the way that, with a few swipes of colorful blush or lipstick, it could literally and figuratively transport a woman from her challenging life to the fantasy of America— a life of leisure and wealth. Marketers realized that if beauty and appearance-related products could become deeply intertwined with symbols of money—and therefore happiness—this experiment could yield a windfall. Some companies, like Estée Lauder, adopted the highly unusual strategy of advertising their products first in Chinese glossy magazines—itself an industry in its infancy—for a full 5 years prior to opening a store in China. Few people could afford these magazines, but by associating themselves with those who could, the company established itself as a symbol of luxury. The strategy seemed to pay off: When Estée Lauder finally launched its flagship boutique in Shanghai in 1993, the demand was so great that rioting ensued.

Others, like L'Oréal, the world's largest cosmetics manufacturer, took a scientific approach, intensively studying the behaviors, rituals, and cultural habits of Chinese self-presentation. This research, begun

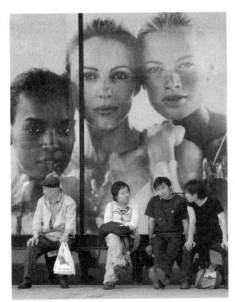

Chinese sit in front of an advertisement for Estée Lauder cosmetics outside a department store in Beijing, Monday, May 17, 2004. The New York-based Estée Lauder, which is to move its Asian headquarters from Singapore to Shanghai, is one of a number of international cosmetics companies trying to tap China's rapidly growing cosmetics market, currently the world's eighth largest.

in 1997, continues today in what has become a global investigation into the self-grooming techniques and preferences of the millions of women who strive to achieve their cultural standards of perfection. For a gigantic company such as L'Oréal, conducting controlled research into such matters is no small feat: An entire division of the company, called Geocosmetics, is staffed with dozens of scientists and analysts, who have meticulously developed a program to best simulate a woman's beauty experience. They began with an innovative idea of videotaping women as they encountered, explored, and applied cosmetics in front of a one-way mirror. "It's what we call an ethnographic approach," Fabrice Aghassian, head of research and development for L'Oréal Paris tells me when we speak on the phone. "For 20 years now, we've been studying consumers in their natural environment—in this case the bathroom—to observe in detail what they do with makeup and how they do it."

And the details are important: In the 2008 report released by Aghassian's Geocosmetics division, researchers noted that it takes, on average, 6 minutes for a Chinese woman to make up her face. Her application techniques include massage and light "tapping" of the facial area—something that can also be observed in Chinese hair salons, as a traditional shampoo can last up to an hour and include massaging of the head, neck, and arms. Scientists can also determine the average number of products worn simultaneously by women from different cultures, as well as the preferred colors and textures.

"In China, there is a significant difference in women's attitudes toward their appearance, depending on age," Aghassian concludes. "Women older than 50 are much less interested in products—they lived for so long with the Communist government, they are not willing to spend on beauty. Women younger than 50 will indulge in cosmetics occasionally. But for women under 30, it is totally different. Beauty for them is a necessity, not a luxury. They are so eager to try new products and invest in their appearance. They also represent 35 percent of the population, or well over 400 million people. So this is our target market."

And target it they have: Five years after entering the Chinese market, L'Oréal recorded sales of $107 million in the country, up 61 percent from the year before. Sales growth in China surpassed all of L'Oréal's other global subsidiaries, with the forecast for the future even rosier.

Having identified their shopper, the next step was to figure out these women's aesthetic preferences. Early on, cosmetics companies found that the primary desire in China's beauty market was neither dramatic eyes nor Angelina lips, but Snow White skin. "Our number one product is Whitestay foundation," says Aghassian. "In Japan, we find that the texture and quality of a facial product is extremely important, but in China, all the focus is on the results. They are not concerned with the ingredients that determine how a product feels if it gives them the look they are seeking." Some of this perhaps is a reflection on the lingering hardships of life in Communist China. In countries with a higher standard of living, quibbling over details like how a product feels or smells makes sense. In a country where the very existence of cosmetics is a relatively new novelty, who cares about the texture if it looks good?

By the 1990s, China's government was encouraging even greater foreign investments, and the country was on the cusp of an economic boom. Young female consumers with growing spending power were hungry to try on an image other than proletariat. The formula was sheer magic: In 1985, China's fledgling beauty industry was valued at a surprisingly high $265 million. Twenty years later, the industry had grown in value to $26.5 billion. After decades of being denied access, everyone—especially women—wanted a piece of the Western pie.

In fact, China's beauty industry is now the eighth-largest market for appearance-driven products in the world, and second in Asia only to Japan. In 2010, China is projected to become number one.[2] Enormous percentages of people's salaries are being spent on body treatments and cosmetics, which are disproportionately expensive when compared to income. The average white-collar job salary in Shanghai, for instance, while higher than most other Chinese cities, is still only 5,000 yuan, or $660 a month. Meanwhile, cosmetics maker Shiseido offers its high-end body cream for 4,000 yuan for a 30-milliliter jar (roughly $480).

Perfection on Sale

As previously mentioned, plastic surgery in China is growing at a faster rate than anywhere else in the world. Along with thin frames and flat stomachs, women are increasingly seeking bigger breasts, more defined noses, longer legs, and rounder eyes. Experts estimate that 3.5 million cosmetic surgery procedures are performed annually in China, and the number continues to rise as the industry grows at a rate of 20 percent each year. In the past 20 years, the country has gone from having zero listed plastic surgeons to more than 7,000 licensed clinics. The country's leading surgeon, Dr. Fushun Ma, says he now performs upward of 10 procedures a day at his clinic. Of course, when you compare the enormity of 3.5 million procedures with the relatively few clinics, you'd have to assume—correctly, as it turns out—that many women who are unable to afford the fees charged by licensed clinics are getting the work done elsewhere, often incurring dangerous risks by signing up for surgery performed by unlicensed practitioners. In fact, China's plastic surgery is, alarmingly, largely unregulated. Dr. Fushun, himself trained and licensed in Canada, reported to *Marie Claire* magazine in 2005 that "every week, 20 or 30 people come into our clinic asking us to correct botched surgery."

The obsession with appearance, even by Western standards, has reached startling heights in a country that just 25 years ago saw the first opening of a cosmetics boutique. But in China, the perfect body equals money, in two ways: Those who can afford cosmetic surgery clearly demonstrate that they are part of China's new, young, monied class. In 2007, there were 345,000 millionaires in the country—an 8 percent increase from the previous year.[3] Procedures such as double eyelid surgery, the most popular operation for women in their twenties and thirties, cost roughly $240 in US dollars; nose shaping runs about $600. Women with either feature—noticeable because it is genetically rare—immediately establish themselves as part of the social elite.

At the same time, looks are money—most women believe they will be able to increase their salaries or land higher-quality jobs if their appearance more closely matches the ideal. It's not just urban legend: Some research (largely propagated by the cosmetic-surgery industry itself) suggests that the women who have undergone plastic surgery generally end up with higher salaries a year later. In a recent survey of college students, one in three believed going under the knife would increase their chances of landing a good job.[4] The competitiveness of the Chinese job market cannot be overlooked—no longer relegated solely to first-tier cities such as Beijing, the economic boom has spread to less-developed cities: In 2006, the average income in second-tier cities increased by 150 percent.[5]

Capitalizing on the boom in cosmetic surgery, in 2004 the government announced the creation of the world's first-ever Miss Plastic Surgery pageant. The criteria for entering were simple: The contestant had to show proof that her fine-tuned physique was courtesy of the miracles of medical science. Though something of a

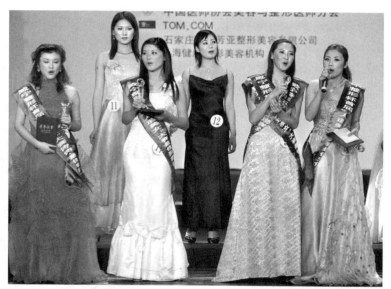

Contestants parade on stage during China's first-ever beauty pageant for women who have had plastic surgery. For the event, held in Beijing on December 18, 2004, competitors had to submit proof that they had undergone surgery. Sponsors included Chinese makers of cosmetic surgery products. The contest included a talent show and evening gown and swimsuit competitions.

spectacle for freaks and gawkers, the pageant was sponsored by several large cosmetic-surgery clinics and attracted several dozen contestants and media attention from around the world. Breast enhancement, jaw sculpting, leg breaking, thigh trimming, and liposuction were just a few of the procedures proudly displayed by the "man-made beauties" (*renzao meinu*) who proudly paraded the catwalks.

Twenty-two-year-old Cao Dandan, a contestant, would have spent $24,000 on her procedures, which required nine separate operations, but she found a way to get them for free: A local hospital was advertising a total body makeover for a woman who would be willing to serve as their cosmetic-surgery spokesperson for the next 5 years. Indeed, many clinics in China are offering free treatments in hopes of word-of-mouth advertising and to build themselves a reputation as a credible clinic for such procedures. Dandan's surgeries ranged from Botox to fat injection in her buttocks; liposuction for her stomach, thighs, and calves; eye and nose surgery; and jaw reshaping. The payoff for Dandan has been substantial: She left her job as a hotel maid and now serves as a tourist guide for wealthy foreigners in Beijing, making three times her previous salary.

For other young women, opting for plastic surgery is less clear—as Mia Lee told me, she recognizes its appeal, but there are other cultural issues that make her hesitate.

Mia's Story

In 21st-century China, beauty is not a natural thing anymore, but a business. If I were to invest in any industry, this is it. Forget about mining, airlines, real estate—beauty is the golden ticket in China.

—MIA LEE, 26, GRADUATE STUDENT, BEIJING

In China, we say there are no ugly women, only lazy women. I believe every Chinese girl can be pretty if she wants to be. I started to think about my own body shape when I was 7 or 8 years old. My school ordered us all to wear uniforms. My size was bigger than other girls, even though I wasn't taller than them. That made me unhappy. Even then, I knew it was not a mark of beauty to look chubby.

Appearance is something women of my generation increasingly focus on. I give myself a C+ compared with Miss Ideal. At 165 centimeters, I am of average height. I've always wished I were taller and my hips were narrower. But at least my naturally C-cup breasts are now all the rage— magazines and billboards everywhere are advertising breast-enhancement procedures.

Like in the United States, celebrity craze is everywhere in China. All celebrities are skinny. The more famous they get, the skinnier they become.

Growing up, the woman I thought (and still think) to be the most beautiful was not a real person but an animation: Lum in the sketch Urusei Yatsura. I like her because she is feminine and physically powerful at the same time. Unlike all the pretty girls in the mass media in China, she is not fragile. She can get pretty violent if she wants. Can Zhang

Ziyi [Crouching Tiger, Hidden Dragon; Memoirs of a Geisha] *beat up boys? I don't think so.*

Young women in China are really judgmental about our celebrities. Rather than put celebrities on a pedestal like goddesses, we see them as okay-looking girls lucky enough to become rich and famous. There is this perception that anyone can make it given the chance.

How do you show that you've "made it"? By spending money on your looks. Cosmetic surgery is growing in China. We even have a Miss Plastic Surgery beauty pageant. I know more than 10 women—and some guys!—who had double eyelid surgery. Myself, I've never made up my mind about plastic surgery. On the one hand, I think it's a woman's right to change her body. On the other, it is considered disrespectful toward your parents to change your face. Still, I have been thinking about getting double eyelid surgery myself.

Staying skinny is all the rage with young women. All the best-selling books last year were about improving your body, instead of literature. For instance, there are all-apple diets where you only eat apples for 5 days. And we have a thousand kinds of herbal teas from various regions of the country that women drink to lose weight. Acupuncture and rubbing coffee beans on your skin are also recommended. There is even one diet where you eat a parasite that grows in your belly! The most extreme example I know of personally is my friend who lived on cucumbers for 15 days.

Young women today care a thousand times more about their looks than 10 years ago. The reform of capitalism

made everything in China a commodity, including wom-
en's bodies. The beauty industry is the fastest-growing
economy in our country. In Chinese, we call a woman's
appearance her number one capital, meaning that's what
she makes her money from. Pretty girls are worth a lot
more in the business world. So money spent on looks is the
best investment a girl can make. She'll earn it all back
later by getting a better job or getting paid more for the job
she already has.

Jobs are so important because the income and lifestyle
gap between the rich and poor is growing. We don't have a
very big middle class. We have some rich people and lots of
poor people. There are people who make in a day what a
peasant family makes in 10 years—and they don't pay a
penny of tax.

I work part-time in an office to help pay for graduate
school. It's an average salary, but I make in 1 week what the
big real estate developers spend on one day's lunch. The ten-
sion between the rich and the poor is enormous. In this kind
of environment, everyone is looking for an edge. So if being
beautiful means you'll make more money, women are not
shy about doing whatever they can to improve their odds."

Waiting for a Backlash

The current obsession with appearance has not come without a
price: In a recent study of Chinese university students, up to 70 percent of women believed they were "too fat," even though their actual

weight fell within the normal range. What gives? "Fatness is subjective in these women's minds," says Sing Lee, MD, director of the Hong Kong Eating Disorders Clinic. Lee tells me that he now sees 25 to 50 times as many female patients for disordered-eating issues than he did 15 years ago. "In one study we did, more than half the women were at normal or below-normal weight, but they were all trying to lose at least 10 pounds."

Thinness, larger breasts, rounder eyes . . . sounds like today's Chinese women are in heavy pursuit of a Westernized ideal. But not so fast. If that is the intent, it may not be an entirely conscious one. Chinese women rarely admit a desire to copy Western aesthetics, says Dr. Fushun: "Usually they just say they believe features such as rounder eyes or higher noses are prettier." In my conversations, the acknowledgment of Western influence tended to break down along generational lines. The women over 40 say yes; they believe that the younger generation is heavily influenced by American advertising, purchasing the shoes, dresses, cosmetics—and now, body shapes—of Barbie. But the younger women adamantly deny this, claiming curvy bosoms simply flatter their otherwise thin frames, and slimness (soft belly or not) has always been a desirable quality. Indeed, already there appears to be a small but growing backlash against appearance alterations that seem too Western: double eyelid surgeries, though still the most popular procedure, declined in 2007. When contestants on China's most popular extreme makeover show were recently asked which famous person they would most like to look like, Asian celebrities, not Caucasian, topped the list (Li Jiaxin, a former Miss Hong Kong, was number one).

This is a marked departure from the trend of the past 10

years, and makes me wonder if China will soon go the way of post-Gorbachev Russia. In the year immediately following Gorbachev's election, Revlon products sold off the shelf so quickly, manufacturers had trouble keeping them in stock; Levi's were the ultimate youth status symbol. "Free market" was a new and exciting term, and everyone wanted a chance to purchase a piece of the American dream. Fast-forward 10 years and Russia's newly wealthy realized that it was foolish to pour money into Western-made goods: Why make America (or Europe) richer? And so Russia began to produce and distribute its own fashion and cosmetics products, cutting out the foreign middleman wherever possible. In China, the real question is whether what is being "purchased" from the West—an actual body type and beauty aesthetic that says money—will morph back into something more traditionally Chinese as their economy begins to rival ours. What would a body ideal best suited for 21st-century China look like? We may find out soon enough.

CHAPTER 5

THE SKINNY STIGMA

The first time I met Sibuele Sibaca she was 18 years old. Dressed in a pink blouse and faded blue jeans, she looked all of about 12—a tiny girl with gigantic brown eyes and long black hair that she wore in a single braid down her back. It was her first trip to America, and she was, quite literally, wide-eyed with amazement at the shops—the shops!—and all the consumerism that consumes our country. She launched into an enthusiastic discussion of her favorite designers, fashion trends, and her aspirations to land a job in the entertainment industry. Her bubbly demeanor, however, belied an underlying sadness. Sibu was an AIDS orphan who lost both of her parents to a disease that is ravaging her nation.

One of the first countries to report incidents of HIV/AIDS, South Africa is also one of the last to openly acknowledge the scope of the pandemic among its people and the means by which it is transmitted, lagging years behind neighboring governments. Lack of information bred fear; fear bred an inclination to ignore, underreport, and decline treatment. All of these factors contributed to a health crisis on a scope never before seen in the 20th century.

Globally, the face of AIDS has shifted dramatically in the first decade of the 21st century. In 1985, HIV infection in sub-Saharan Africa affected men and women equally. According to a 2007 United Nations AIDS report, 61 percent of the HIV positive in sub-Saharan Africa are women—the highest population of infected women in the world. Moreover, the South African Department of Health estimated in 2006 that one in three pregnant women was HIV positive. The numbers weigh even more heavily against young adult women: Among South Africans ages 18 to 24, women are three times more likely than men to be HIV positive.

Women in South Africa are particularly vulnerable to contracting the disease for a number of reasons: lack of sex education and prevention, cultural attitudes toward their gender, and an exceptionally high rate of female rape among them.

To further complicate matters, AIDS—a taboo disease in almost every culture—is especially stigmatized in South Africa. Thus, even when people suspect they may be ill, they rarely seek medical attention because of the shame and social ostracizing they fear will ensue. This paranoia is not unfounded—a recent study revealed that 1 in 10 HIV-positive South Africans who admitted the illness to their families was met with swift hostility.[1] Only recently have the majority of AIDS victims begun to aggressively seek medical help, and by the time they do, the disease has usually progressed to an advanced stage.

It is not surprising, then, that in South Africa there are well over

1.1 million AIDS orphans, a number expected to surpass 3 million by 2010. These children, like Sibu, are left to fend for themselves; if they are the eldest of the surviving family, they are often expected to assume the role of parent and raise their younger siblings. Without community support, every day becomes a fight for survival. Boys may find employment in manual labor. Too often for female AIDS orphans, their bodies are the only commodities they have to sell, and so they do. Eventually they, too, become infected with the virus, and the AIDS cycle continues.

In such an environment, it's not surprising that people have become fearful and suspicious of those who are suspected to be ill. It starts with the death or mysterious disappearance of a friend or relative; then the rumors begin to swirl. Who will be next? Is the rest of the family sick too? How can you tell? The most obvious way to assess someone's health begins with appearance, and when it comes to AIDS, the telltale physical symptoms of infection are unmistakable: body rashes, a loss of healthy skin color, and dramatic, unexplained weight loss. "In South Africa, whether in rural regions or the poor urban communities, people have come to equate thinness with illness, and rightly so," says Mieke Faber, PhD, the director of the Nutritional Intervention Residential Unit of the Medical Research Council in Tygerberg, South Africa.

If thinness is associated with illness, does the opposite hold true as well? Faber studied the relationship between body size and perceptions of wellness in her native country.[2] She found that larger figures for South African women were considered attractive—and the number-one criterion for attractiveness was good health. In the population she studied, 41 percent of the women were overweight and another 30 percent were medically obese. Despite these facts, only 2 percent of the overweight women considered themselves too heavy; only one in three of the obese group felt this was the case. Moreover, even among those who believed they were too heavy, virtually none expressed a desire to lose weight through dieting.

There are two health-related factors at work here, says Faber: First is the immediate connection that communities, especially the men, make between plumpness and good health. "From the male perspective, a fuller figure for the wife is an indication that she is being looked after," she explains. If the woman is married, her girth indicates to others that she is being treated right by her husband. It is also a sign of her husband's relative economic power: The bigger the woman, the more money her husband must have for food, and food, in parts of South Africa, is still a scarce and expensive commodity. Food, says Faber, "plays a very important role in showing wealth" and also less tangible qualities such as happiness and a strong community, as it "plays the central role in everything from weddings to funerals."

If South Africa were America, public health authorities would undoubtedly bemoan such a burgeoning obesity crisis. Though South Africa does not track obesity in the same way we do in the United States, evidence suggests that by Western measurements, a significant proportion of the population is overweight. But because weight loss (in addition to simply being naturally thin) is associated with HIV/AIDS, many heavier women don't attempt to shed pounds, even if, medically speaking, it would be advisable to do so. Says Faber, "Most women in our research felt that losing weight was a sign of ill health, and moreover would unfavorably change their status within their community." Anecdotally, this idea was supported by the women I spoke with, regardless of their actual body size.

Sibu's Story

The other kids teased me, then they feared me. Being thin is no great thing in South Africa.

—SIBU SIBACA, 24,
ACCOUNTS MANAGER, JOHANNESBURG

I was only 9 when my mom died. I was 16 when my father passed away. I didn't know until both of them were gone that they'd died from AIDS. My father was a pastor; my mother taught at the local school. We were middle class by American standards, but we never wanted for anything, my brother and I. We had a nice house, cars, a big garage. Education was important to my parents, so I took school quite seriously. But for all that education, I never learned about AIDS.

I am not the typical body type for a black South African. I am "like a bird," as my family used to say—all limbs, no curves. For years, my mother tried to fatten me up, giving me more food, encouraging me to eat more. In South Africa, thinness is not a desirable quality. I never looked like the other children, which concerned my mother a great deal. Mainly what I remember from being a young girl was trying to fit in.

As hard as it was when my parents were alive, it was

when they passed away that things got really hard. I found out they'd died of HIV/AIDS through the gossip mill. As we say in South Africa, good news travels fast, but bad news travels faster. People started to talk, giving me funny looks. I caught wind of what people were saying, and I confronted my brother. I'd read about AIDS in a biology book at school, but it wasn't something the teacher discussed, and it never crossed my mind that this disease could take away anyone I knew, let alone my parents. There is such a stigma to AIDS—even talking about it is taboo. As a consequence, it has spread throughout the country like crazy while people look the other way. It's as if by not saying the word you can somehow make it disappear.

My brother admitted that our parents had died of AIDS. My father apparently told him that he was infected, but he thought he could "protect" me by not saying anything. I was shocked and really hurt. In South Africa, there is a gender bias in how males and females are treated and allowed to behave. Women are told nothing, and they are supposed to stay home and be proper. Men talk about the "important" stuff. That's fine, I suppose, but if the men are out acting crazy, they will bring the disease back into the home and there is nothing that women can do about it. They don't even know what it is.

At age 16, I became an AIDS orphan. The emotional part of losing both parents was numbing, but worse was the way I lost friends overnight. Girlfriends I used to be close to started whispering about my family, about the fact I was skinny and that could mean I had AIDS too. I was so angry, but there was nothing I could do to stop all the gossip. At first I tried so hard to eat more, to get bigger, to show I was healthy. But that's not my body type, and I eventually decided I couldn't change my body just to prove a point.

In my head, I knew it was almost impossible that I'd contracted the disease since I understood how it was transmitted and I never had risky sex with boys in school. But I started doubting myself when everyone in my community began ignoring me, ostracizing me. Parents wouldn't let their daughters hang out with me anymore. I had already lost my parents; now I felt totally alone.

Girls learn much of their information about body image from their mothers, but even then, it is less common for South Africans to discuss topics about the body. Partly I think because in rural areas there is some shame in your body—certain groups practice routine "virginity checks" on girls, which can make them afraid to ask questions.

But as a general rule, the preferred body size for women is larger than in the United States. Not fat, but definitely not the thin look of American models. My mother had what would be considered the ideal body shape for a South African woman. She was big and curvy, and I remember wishing I looked more like she did. I was too young when she died to have any meaningful conversations with her about beauty and such, but I do remember being horrified at how much weight she was losing when she got sick. I knew it was because she was ill; I just didn't know it was AIDS.

In South Africa, you cannot just "lose weight" the way you can in America by dieting. The minute you start shedding pounds, people will start asking questions out of concern for your health. It is not something people applaud. I think this is slowly changing, especially since there is ironically also an obesity concern in parts of the country. The more educated people become about AIDS, the less afraid they are about something like dieting for health reasons. They realize losing weight is not necessarily an indication that you have a disease they can "catch."

I see more women going to the gym now than 5 years ago, but it's still not popular like it is in Western countries. This will always be a country that praises its women for being bigger—big equals wealth in South Africa; it means you come from a family that can afford to feed you; and it traditionally means men will pay more for you in dowry because you look healthier.

How do I know things have not changed? Because I still cannot go clothes shopping and find dresses that fit a smaller woman's body. In these shops, everything is tailored to the bigger woman. Like women all over the world, I am not 100 percent satisfied with my body, but I have learned to make peace with not fitting the South African ideal. I am not terribly happy about being 24 years old and looking like I'm still 12, but this is what I have been given. I have a boyfriend who appreciates my smaller size and compliments me on my figure.

Today, I have a good job as an accounts manager for a mar-keting company. I am making a life for myself despite what I have been through. I may have lost my family, but I will not become another one of the sad AIDS orphan statistics.

Beyond the influence of the AIDS epidemic, other factors promote the idea that bigger women are healthier, wealthier, and more successful. "In South Africa, particularly rural parts of the country, women get their information about nutrition and healthy body size from their mothers, grandmothers, older women in the community," notes Faber. Body ideals are passed directly from one generation to the next. "When you are surrounded by other women who are overweight but also respected in the community, you become comfortable thinking that being overweight is actually normal." Moreover, "there are a significant number of black women in Parliament who are overweight, and one could argue that younger black women associate success with a heavier body shape."

Additional studies validate Faber's findings. In a 2005 report published in the *South African Journal of Clinical Nutrition*, researcher Tanie Puoane[3] found that even among health workers, the perception that "big is beautiful" is dominant.

"Experience shows that thinner people die sooner in South Africa," she explains when I reach her by phone. "It is not some aesthetic pulled out of the air or mythology that makes Africans prefer fuller body shapes—it is borne out time and time again when you look at life expectancy and health statistics. Bigger bodies are perceived to be more desirable because people equate size with good health."

In Puoane's study of 44 female health-care workers in South

Africa, only two of them were a medically healthy weight; the rest were overweight or obese. When asked to describe the ideal female body, a moderately overweight figure (women with a body mass index of about 27) was consistently preferred. The study participants associated this plump figure with dignity, community respect, confidence, beauty, and wealth in addition to good health. A separate study in the *Journal of Medical Marketing*[4] observed that selling a South African audience on the notion of weight loss products was an uphill battle due to the general perception that "obesity is being seen to denote health and freedom from HIV infection, whereas weight loss is perceived to indicate HIV infection. This further entrenches perceptions that obesity is healthy and . . . suggests that medical marketers must carefully design their strategies for marketing medicine for obesity-related diseases in regions with high HIV infections to avoid being accused of trying to benefit from the interaction of both epidemics."

So "big is beautiful" thrives in South Africa in part because it is the clearest physical evidence that a woman is free from a deadly disease. But hand in hand with this understanding is the implication that a larger body is also a sign of economic prosperity.

Obesity researchers have found time and time again, in South Africa and other countries where food is a precious commodity, that higher weight is equated with greater wealth, and greater wealth with better health.

In October 2007, *Freakonomics* author Stephen J. Dubner highlighted the findings of two female economists in his weekly *New York Times* blog.[5] The researchers, Anne Case, PhD, and Alicia Menendez, PhD, had spent several months in South Africa measuring the economic variables that influence the body shapes and size preferences of the country's women. Their findings, illustrated in quantitative charts and mathematical equations, boil down to this: Women of higher socioeconomic status in South Africa are statistically more likely to be obese than women of lower socioeconomic status. The economists suggested that this fact directly reflects wealthier women's ability to access food. The flip side is the subsequent cultural expectation that larger women are likely to be richer, because size is a by-product of money. In this way, a fuller figure comes to represent higher social status, which in turn inspires other local women to "admire larger body sizes."

The framework for Case and Menendez's study was straightforward: They collected data from women with a wide variety of body sizes, measuring their height, weight, and body mass index. Participants were then asked to look at a series of simple illustrations (devoid of any personal characteristics or facial expressions) of women's body shapes, ranging from underweight to obese. When the overweight or obese women in the group were asked to choose an image that best matched their own body size, they consistently selected a body shape that was *heavier* than their actual figure. Moreover, when asked how they felt about the body shape they selected, the women overwhelmingly expressed satisfaction and happiness with it. This finding is in direct contrast with similar studies that have been conducted in the United States and that have found that American women, who generally express less satisfaction with the state of their bodies, also tend to overestimate their actual size. And their emotional reaction to being a larger size is predominantly negative.

Case and Menendez concluded from their research that for

South African women, "perceptions of an 'ideal' female body are larger than men's perceptions of the 'ideal' male body, and individuals with larger 'ideal' body images are significantly more likely to be obese."

Black and White

Wealth, social status, and health are three reasons that South African women favor a heavier body size. A fourth, more complicated reason can be traced to the historic tensions between blacks and white colonials in South Africa's violent past. Beginning in the mid-17th century, the black tribes of South Africa were consistently engaged in conflict with the European colonizers. The Portuguese arrived first in the early 16th century, followed by the Dutch, and in the early 19th century, the British. The clash between blacks and whites in South Africa is a well-documented history of racial oppression, abuse, and cultural misunderstanding.

For centuries, the mark of beauty for South Africa's black women was larger lower bodies. Buttocks, hips, legs—these were the focus of local fashion and the most admired areas of a woman's figure. In fact, the Ndebele tribe's fashion dictated that women wear large beaded hoops around their waists and legs, called *golwani*. These garments were then stuffed with rubber to enhance the apparent size of the wearer's bottom and legs. "Among black natives, large buttocks and thighs were considered a sign of womanliness," says Carolyn Martin Shaw, PhD, a professor of anthropology at the University of California, Santa Cruz. Often likened to "rolls of fat," the *golwani* was a must-have accessory for young women, especially important for dancing in local festivals.

Much of the dancing itself was designed to feature women's volup-tuous hips and thighs. "Large buttocks were the focal point of cele-bratory dances," says Shaw. "These dances required women to turn their backsides to the audience and show off their fantastic muscle control by contracting their buttocks in rhythm with the music."

Traditions such as these, which the Ndebele and Zulu tribes con-tinued to practice to varying degrees throughout British occupation, helped the black community maintain their identity despite growing oppression during colonial rule and postindependence, when the last ties to British government were finally severed in 1960.

Yet black South Africans still suffered under apartheid for another 3 decades, until in April 1994, the country held its first-ever universal suffrage general elections, symbolically transitioning the country from a polarized republic to a fledgling democracy. Blacks and whites voted side by side, and the balance of power shifted toward the major-ity, which was, by a ratio of four to one, the black population. Now that the political interests of black South Africans were represented, social equality was mandated. But what was written on paper was clearly more complicated in reality. True economic equality would take years, given the institutionalized disparity that existed for so long between races. In 1995, the majority of businesses in South Africa were owned by whites. Eighty percent of low-wage, unskilled jobs were held by blacks. How could a group that had been held down for so long attain the financial freedom they wanted? What was the fastest route to securing better jobs, higher paychecks, and the next rung on the economic ladder?

Enter the most visible collateral for trading one lifestyle for another: the body. As you would imagine, the white European population in South Africa subscribed to European fashion trends and body shape preferences. Black culture—once a source of pride—was now a very obvious and symbolic barrier between poor blacks and wealthy whites. A heavier body may have indicated wealth in the black community, but the same did not hold true even in the poorest white communities.

So perhaps when a group of researchers studied the body images and attitudes of young black women in South Africa in the late 1990s,[6] the results shouldn't have been surprising. And yet no one expected their findings to be so dramatic. For several months, researcher Julie Seed, PhD, and her colleagues from Northumbria University in the United Kingdom collected data on the eating habits of black female college students in rural areas of South Africa. This population was selected for their higher level of potential financial success, an estimation based on their pursuit of a university diploma. But education and money were not enough for these women to feel as though they were on a level playing field with their white peers; they also felt compelled to match them in appearance. "At least 45 percent of the black students we studied showed some form of disordered eating," says Seed. In fact, Zulu women were characterized as having the fastest-growing rate of eating disorders of any community in the country. "Considering that this culture consistently valued bigness over thinness for years, and [it was one] in which generous proportions were historically seen as a sign of wealth and beauty, this was an alarming discovery."

It's ironic that the collapse of apartheid appears to have triggered a radical shift in body ideals. "Prior to the end of apartheid in 1994, there were no documented cases of eating disorders within the black

South African community," says Seed. "But post-apartheid, women in the black community saw the possibilities for better jobs and wages—so long as they could fit into the white-dominated work world of higher-paying jobs. In other words, being more like a white person would increase their odds of success." Looking "big" was a flashback to black South Africans' past, Seed points out, and nothing in that past would help young, educated women land the corporate, traditionally white-person's job in the future.

Taking Back the Motherland

After spending half a decade trying to mold themselves into the white South Africans' body ideals and aesthetics, black women began to renounce the presumption that they had to look "white" to be treated equally and gain access to the same educational and economic opportunities. Some of this reemergence of black aesthetics and culture can be attributed to the rise in the number of black South Africans holding high positions in government, media, and business, as well as the strategic decisions they made to cater to an increasingly affluent black clientele. In Johannesburg, for instance, Litha Nkombisa launched Joburg City Auto in 1993. It was the first black-owned car dealership in the city's history. Making a shrewd business decision about the kind of image he wanted to project, Nkombisa and his partners decided to sell only BMWs. South Africa's blacks, he said, deserved the best car. In his first month, Nkombisa sold 42 BMWs, a record for the city. The secret to success, says Nkombisa, who calls Nelson Mandela his role model, is talking to the customers in the way they are accustomed to, not trying to impress them by acting "white." The new South Africa is one where the people running the show actually look like the people in the audience. When your colleagues and bosses are black, fitting into the white physical ideal is considerably less vital.

But as precedents were set from the top down, they were also created from the bottom up. In the years after apartheid, black South Africans "began to be proud of themselves, because before that they were made to believe in the European style of beauty," said Jabu Stone, one of South Africa's leading hairstylists known for his skill in styling traditional African locks.[7] Sociologists note that one of the initial signs of the resurgence in black pride could be found in the boom of black hair salons and street stalls for black hairstyling in the late 1990s. As much as body shape is an indicator of black culture, so too are dreadlocks, plaits, and braids.

"People (are) starting to be themselves and to be proud of who they are and to realize that their culture is what they can sell to the outside world," said Stone. "Natural is here to stay. Because of the apartheid era, people were taught that to be black was a sin. All I'm saying is forget that. Let's go back to who we are."

Perhaps one of the most telling signs that times are changing can be found in the number of previously white-owned beauty salons for white-only customers that are now either catering to black clientele or have been completely taken over by black owners who charge as much as one-tenth the average South African's monthly salary for traditional African hairstyles. These days, looking "authentically black" will cost you. And perhaps therein lies a telling secret: When personal appearance products, services, or experiences begin to charge slightly more than the average person can comfortably pay, it can become a "luxury service" or high-end trend. And for people looking to scale social and economic ladders, such goods quickly become very desirable. Think of the Starbucks effect: For (at least) $3 a pop, your morning coffee can buy you not only a fancy caffeine jolt, but the feeling of being included in an elite, higher-income circle.

Under certain circumstances, that would make you a sucker. But under others, such as in South Africa, inflating the cost of looking "black" has had the effect of making it socially desirable to be a true African, and has encouraged young women to embrace their bodies. Along with an appreciation for black hair and beauty products, consumers are making it known that a fuller, thicker figure with a pronounced derriere is the preferred aesthetic. If South Africa's European-based clothing stores cannot accommodate this shape, black women simply don't have to spend their money there.

Khanyi's Story

There is a renaissance movement afoot in South Africa. Women are remembering all the reasons we have to be proud of our full, curvy figures.

—KHANYI MAGUBUNE, 29,
RADIO PRESENTER, JOHANNESBURG

For too long, the black woman's body has been under attack; in cities like Joburg, you see black women trying to look white-slim. And black women bleaching their skin to look whiter. It's time to take our bodies back. The black South African woman is celebrated for her big buns and big hips and big bosom. This is what makes a woman beautiful.

Body confidence in the black community has always been high. I am comfortable with my body; it is not perfect, but my mother always told me that what matters is not whether you have the "best" whatever, but that whatever you have, you make sure that you put your best self forward.

My mother died from complications due to surgery when I was 20. My father died when I was 11. So I am on my own, as many young people in South Africa are. I had to grow up fast, but it's made me passionate, feisty, and outspoken on the issues that matter most to me.

One of those issues is the resurgence of black pride in my country. Black women are realizing we don't have to be just one thing, or one mind in order to make an impact. There are many ways my generation can express themselves and we are: This is the African Renaissance Movement you can see, where women are changing their names back from European to more traditionally African ones, and getting their hair done into dreadlocks at one of the many new salons that specialize only in traditional hair. We also have the Black Economic Empowerment movement, the women we also dub "black diamonds" because they like flashy things—fancy cars, expensive clothes. They don't believe there is a future in the African Renaissance Movement because it is not economically profitable. We'll see about that.

I consider myself a member of the Creative Movement, women who are artists and writers and poets and thinkers, who wear bright colors and beads and express ourselves through our vibrant outfits. The best part about it all, though, is that women are realizing they can be whatever they want. And that pertains to body size too. You can be big or small—but big will always be what blacks here consider beautiful. Myself, would you believe I was actually a contestant briefly on South Africa's version of The Biggest Loser?! *I've always been a big person. I thought, should I now try to be different?*

So I guess it's no surprise to anyone that I was kicked off the first show. My body is what it is. I even gained weight on the show! It's just a different culture for blacks—even the words we choose to describe our body reveal this: When a guy says, "Yo, that girl is fit, man!" what he means by "fit" is that she is built like a brick house. I think in America, you say "fit" and it means something very different!

Black women are not going to change their body shape to accommodate anyone's culture but our own. If something is going to change, it will have to be others bending to our ideals.

One of the first apparel companies to take note of the black consumer spending power was Levi Strauss. Levi's, the ubiquitous symbol of youth and pop culture, have always been popular among South African teens. But the company began to notice a drop in sales 5 years ago, and so they conducted a survey to better understand their black female customers. They learned that while young women said they liked the brand, most felt that they couldn't fit into the company's jeans, or that the cut of the jeans—modeled on Caucasian figures—wouldn't flatter their bodies.

"Young African women are increasingly proud of their body shape and are celebrating it in fashion," said Levi's South African managing director in an interview. "There is a marked confidence in African identity compared to 5 or 10 years ago, and while young Africans are making use of international brands, they want to maintain their sense of being African."

With this information in hand, what would you—as a clothing company and universally recognized fashion icon—do? There are certain high-end designers (Gucci and Prada come to mind) who refuse to cut their clothing for fuller figures, maintaining that their fashions are designed for women with a certain look. But Levi's South Africa office saw a tremendous sales opportunity: They could tailor the cut and sizing of their product to the body shape of a new consumer. Marketers scrambled to figure out how best to sell to the new black South African woman: educated and proud, with a penchant for beauty and an ability to spend millions more every year than she could a decade ago.

And so Levi's introduced a new line: EVA jeans, which the company describes as "designed to have more fabric and stretch in the seat, with a curved waistband which is higher at the back and lower in the front for a flattering fit around the waist." In an interview with one of South Africa's leading business publications, marketing director Debbie Gebhardt described the jeans and their growing popularity within other markets: "Shape rather than sizing was the problem. We had to create a new hip-to-waist ratio. Developed for the local market, we now realize that Levi's EVA has global appeal. Stars like Beyoncé, Shakira, and J-Lo have destigmatized curvy bodies and popularized 'bootyliciousness.' There are limited options for women with this body shape, and the success of Levi's EVA proves this."

When Levi's made the decision to reach out to the young black population's perception of the ideal body, they hit pay dirt. While Gebhardt wouldn't release the actual figures, she did say that the company has experienced a "tremendous increase in sales." Given that 80 percent of South Africa is black, I'd say that's quite a large increase. It's even bigger when you consider that a whopping one in four pairs of jeans sold in South Africa belongs to this brand alone.

It is with a bit of irony that I learn EVA may soon launch in the United States. "Black and Latina women in America have more money to spend, and less patience when it comes to looking for clothes that fit their curvier figures," says Gebhardt. "We expect EVA jeans to have a similar success with this market."

In South Africa, EVA is held up as an example of the power of the almighty rand—consumers with money to spend are consumers you want, but with that money also comes the power to decide where and how to use it. A savvy company will listen to what these consumers are clamoring for and adapt their merchandise accordingly. In South Africa, clothing companies better get ready for a roller coaster of product-adapting. From bigger bodies to a thin Euro aesthetic and back to full figures once more, there could hardly be another place on Earth that better makes this point: Nothing in the world of female body ideals ever stays flat for long.

CHAPTER 6

A PRECURSOR TO GLOBALIZATION

L ong before globalization became the buzzword of the 21st century—before Microsoft began outsourcing tech jobs to India or Starbucks set up shop in Moscow—one American company saw the benefits in global expansion. Coca-Cola—a company whose products, packaging, television jingles, graphics, and flavors are virtually ingrained in every American's brain—began exporting its iconic bottles in the beginning of the 20th century.

Today Coca-Cola can be found in 144 countries, in more than a dozen flavors. Coke product sales made the company nearly $16 billion in 2006 alone. Those who drink it, unwittingly or not, become part of the Coca-Cola image, one that mirrors American pop culture and its love of music, clothes, sports, cars, and generation-specific vocabulary. At home and abroad, Coca-Cola has historically been equated with youth and its accompanying "cool" factor.

But when the distinctive 10-ounce glass Coca-Cola bottle arrived in Jamaica for the first time in the 1930s, it acquired a meaning far different than the all-American beverage. It became, in a relatively short period of time, a metaphor of feminine beauty on the Caribbean island. The imported bottle's shape, with its small bubble at the top, tapered middle, and wide base, was remarkably similar to the female silhouette aspired to by Jamaican women—the large-bottomed, curvy-bosomed woman with ample flesh padding either side of her narrowed waist, an ideal left over from Jamaica's African heritage. The term *Coca-Cola–bottle shape* was quickly integrated into the popular lexicon as the description for a woman with the perfect body. Though there is no way of knowing exactly when the phrase was coined, it's easy to imagine men relaxing in a bar after work, mixing their bottles of soda with shots of alcohol and perhaps noting, through a pleasant haze, that the glass bottle in their hands was not unlike the shape of an attractive woman.

A decade after its debut, the popularity of the soft drink—and its imagery—had spread across the Caribbean, giving birth to such songs as the Jamaican calypso tune "Rum + Coca-Cola." An instant hit on the island, the song became an international favorite after being picked up by American radio stations. In fact, it eventually climbed the charts to become the third best-selling single of the 1940s. The Coca-Cola–bottle-shape craze peaked in the 1990s, when reggae artist Simpleton wrote a song that topped the charts, called, naturally, "Coca-Cola Shape":

> *Coca-Cola woman . . . mermaid body*
> *She arrives at the dance*
> *Making a grand entrance*
> *I get all excited to get closer to her . . .*

The song's popularity lasted throughout the '90s and is still played in clubs today—a testament, perhaps, to the body ideal that's still going strong.

The Coca-Cola–bottle shape as a reference to the ideal woman's body has persisted in Jamaican culture for decades. As with many developing countries, large body size, particularly for women, is an important indicator of status and wealth; heavier women are also considered more attractive. Thinness is pitied. "In Jamaica, keeping slim has antisocial connotations," says Elisa Sobo, a professor of anthropology at San Diego State University. "Ideally, relatives provide for each other, sharing money and food. Because kin feed each other, no one ever becomes thin."

Psychologist and body image researcher Gail Ferguson, PhD, who was born in Jamaica and now resides in the United States, echoes this sentiment: "I was home last month for the first time in several years. And the very first thing my mother-in-law said when she saw me was, 'Come, let me see if you've gained any weight.' And when she concluded that I had, she was quite pleased. Imagine an American mother-in-law saying that to her son's wife!" (Ferguson added that her own discomfort with this exchange—something she would have thought nothing of 10 years ago—was a sign to her that she was becoming "Westernized.")

In Jamaica, women proudly discuss weight gain—the implication being, if you are well loved and successful in life, you will develop a fuller figure. In this way, size is seen as a social barometer—and weight loss is a sign of neglect. In fact, the ultimate insult is to tell a woman she has a "*Diet* Coke shape," since, until recently, Diet Coke only came in cans—and cans don't have curves. The Jamaican Creole term for a thin woman is *mauger*, which roughly translates as "meager and powerless, and lacking in social commitment from her community."[1] Calling a woman fat, however, is far from disparaging. "It is not an insult as it is in the US," says Ferguson. "Fatness is not universally seen as a bad thing."

The popularity of a curvy body hearkens back to Jamaica's African slave heritage, and a general preference among many African cultures for a fleshier female physique. It also happens to look extraordinary in motion on the dance floor, which is where, on any given night, you will find the largest percentage of young Jamaican adults. Fifty years ago, it was calypso music. Today, the dance halls are crowded with twentysomethings pressed body to body as deejays play a mix of reggae and hip-hop, songs generally about women, sex, and the good life. From midnight until dawn, you will find young women and men dancing in next to nothing, performing hip-shaking, pelvic-gyrating moves in rhythm to the pulsing beat. "The curves of a Jamaican woman's body are essential for this kind of dancing," says Sobo, "and dancing is central to community life."

Accessorizing the body with short skirts and tight tops accentuates the curves. In an affirmation of Jamaican women's absolute body confidence, notes one dance-hall regular I spoke with, "It matters not a bit whether she is the thinnest or heaviest woman in the room—Jamaicans in the dance hall will wear whatever the latest trend is, as long as it shows as much of their flesh as possible."

In April 2007, during one of Jamaica's many popular carnivals at Beach J'ouvert, the deejay of the ceremonies called out to the crowd to turn up their enthusiasm. "To all the women who know they have a Coca-Cola–bottle shape," he shouted, "bring yourselves backstage and get painted Coca-Cola colors!" A flock of drink-happy, body-confident women filed behind the screen, later to reemerge in red-and-white body paint for a raucous, sexually blunt dance-off with the deejay.

The majority of dancing takes place in the dance halls, where the common way for a man to "ask" for a dance is to gyrate his pelvis up close to a woman's backside, and place his hands on her hips. If a woman begins to move her hips in rhythm with the man behind her, it is a sign that she has accepted his request for a dance. "The dance-hall culture has spawned music and movements heavily sexual in nature, and favorable to a curvy Coca-Cola–bottle-shape body," says Sobo.

Of course, the full-figured woman was iconicized in Jamaica long before dance halls existed. But the relationship between the preferred body shape and popular forms of dance is nevertheless essential to understanding the pervasiveness of the Jamaican body ideal. "It's a chicken-versus-egg question," says Ferguson. "Certainly you can say that Jamaican music has helped change our ideas about what type of physical appearance is socially acceptable. It may not have created the body ideal, but it reflects the reality of women's bodies and perpetuates, through song and dance, a certain body preference."

Enthusiasm for fuller figures can also be traced to Jamaican folk beliefs about the body, particularly the notion of "vital fluids." Believed to be the fluids of vitality and fertility—necessary to make and live life—it was traditionally thought that these fluids flow through healthy men and women, leaving the body literally bursting with life at the seams. "Think of a ripe fruit, or a camel's hump, or an aloe plant after the rain," says Sobo. "They are in good health and full of these vital fluids." To be full figured is to be full of vital life liquid in Jamaica, a concept that so permeates society that men will refer to teenage girls as "soon ripe," and reference harvesting analogies when talking about having sex with "ripe" women.

Marcia's Story

After having three children, I lost so much weight my mother-in-law was embarrassed. She worried people would think her son was not caring enough for his wife.

—MARCIA ANDERSON, 53,
RETIRED SCHOOLTEACHER, JAMAICA

The first time I remember actively investigating my body and the anatomical difference between girls and boys, I was about 9 years old. I had just barely started to grow breasts, and my closest cousin, who was a month younger, was developing at a much faster pace than I was. This bothered me, as I was quite skinny as a child, and incredibly self-conscious about it. I don't know why, but for as long as I was aware of my body, I was also aware that bigger women were considered more attractive. Some parents even gave their children appetite stimulants to help them fill out faster. I remember one photo taken at the beach from my preteen years. I showed my bones all too well, and I was embarrassed by it.

In my early teens, I started following the current fashions in Jamaica, some based on European ideas, but always modified for the Jamaican body. I was aware of how various styles accentuated the waist in relation to the bust and hips. Blouses and skirts for girls were not tight—many of us wore what is called a "hobble skirt" [an ankle-length garment loose at the hips and bunched tight below the knees, inhibiting walking; hence the term hobble]—but it was most important to wear a tight belt to give the body the proper proportion of the Coca-Cola–bottle shape.

I don't remember my mother ever talking about her body, but she showed her body confidence in other ways— she'd played sports in school, and worked for years as a gym teacher. I have a photograph of her riding a horse in a way considered "unladylike" [i.e., Western-style, legs straddling the horse] and other pictures of her wearing pants long before this was an acceptable style for women. So she was in some ways very modern in her thinking about the body, but talking about it with her children was out of the question. When it came time to learn about the birds and bees, she gave me a booklet. There was no q&a session afterward.

I grew up in rural Jamaica, in the Santa Cruz Mountains. Television had only just come to the country when I was a child, and certainly cinemas were few and far between where I lived. So Hollywood really had no influence on my early ideas about women's bodies. In my teenage years, as I realized the importance of proportion between a woman's hips, waist, and bust, I concluded that my own hips were not well shaped. They were too "low," as they marked the beginning of my thighs, rather than the end of my waist. The bright side to this was that I realized I had enviably shapely legs. I would never have my cousin's cleavage, but I'd filled out enough to proudly show off my body in a bikini at the pool.

One thing I didn't give much thought to was my rear end. Out of sight, out of mind, as they say! But later I realized that boys had taken great note, even if I hadn't, of its shape and dimensions. Most boys and men got their ideas about women's bodies from publications that had nothing to do with fashion or clothes, if you know what I mean. And the daily newspaper cartoons featured women with enormous bottoms, bulbous breasts, and very prominent thighs. When a man found a woman's body to be pleasing, he would call her "fat" or "beef." I was flattered to be called both.

It was while taking a dance class (there were no dance halls back then) that I came to realize the importance attached to the buttocks. The instructor put us through a series of exercises to shape the buttocks, and special attention was paid to whether we were developing our bottoms properly from class to class.

Several years later, when I was 18, hot pants came into fashion, and I sewed myself several pairs. Suddenly, my bum was of ultimate importance. I discovered discreetly displaying my body through certain clothes brought me more than a few compliments, and so I began paying more attention to my shape. I liked my full figure—I grew up *thinking chubby people were the nicest, since many of my loving relatives were plump.*

I married young and had three children in the first 4 years. After the third, I did need to lose a bit of the baby fat. I never liked to diet, so instead I prayed for it to go away. Eventually it did, and I kept it off for 20 years and two more children. In fact, I lost so much weight as to alarm my mother-in-law. She was embarrassed, and worried people would think her son was not caring enough for his wife. To us, a thin person was an underfed person, a testimony to poverty. I remember when Twiggy became famous—Jamaicans found it ludicrous. It just goes to show, you can't please everyone, so it's best to focus on pleasing God and your conscience first!

For my generation, the concern was less body size, more skin color and hair texture. Black pride had yet to come to Jamaica, and the aftermath of slavery still made some upper-class people wish for whiter features. They were also less favorably disposed to being significantly overweight, while on the grassroots level, amplitude spilling out of a skimpy top, at the midriff and below, was regarded as sexy and a come-on.

Today, at 53, I am not entirely happy with my body. I have lost my shapely legs. I have folds and bulges in the wrong places. I need to lose about 50 pounds for optimal health. But I still recall fondly the pleasures of having a Coca-Cola–bottle shape, and knowing the boys found me "fat," in the very best sense of the word.

Pop Pressure

Like any ideal body, a perfect Coca-Cola–bottle shape is something to strive for. But the discrepancy between a Jamaican woman's actual size and the physique to which she aspires is far less dramatic than, say, the gap between an American size 2 and a size 14. Psychologists and sociologists believe that this achievability contributes to the unusual staying power of Jamaica's "perfect body" ideal,[2] because it elevates body confidence for most women.

According to researchers, a woman's body confidence is largely determined by three variables: her actual size, the size she *wishes* to be, and the size that is preferred by the "elite" members of pop society (think Hollywood stars and boldface tabloid names).[3] "Girls have a higher self-esteem when there is greater agreement between these elements," says Ferguson.

In Jamaica, because actual and ideal bodies are fairly closely aligned, women are confident about the way they look. And that confidence, in turn, helps strengthen the existing ideal, so the pressure to alter one's body is less urgent. "The main difference between the Coca-Cola–bottle-shape ideal and the Barbie ideal put forth in the US is that the Coca-Cola–bottle shape is accessible—you don't have to change your corpus to get it," says Eileen Anderson-Fye, EdD, a medical anthropologist at Case Western Reserve University in Cleveland who has studied the Coca-Cola–bottle-shape ideal in San Andres, Belize. (These similar body ideals between countries are attributed to proximity—Belize is a neighboring country just west of Jamaica—and their shared African heritage.) "It is a very American belief that you can achieve anything as an individual, and shaping the individual body is an extension of that belief. Working with young women with eating disorders in the US, there is an absence of the notion that there are genetic or physical limitations to the changes you can make to your body."

In Anderson-Fye's research, she interviewed teenage girls in San Andres about their body ideals and body image. In response to her question about pursuing the Coca-Cola ideal, one girl told her, "God gave me this body as it is; I can't change it, and even if I did, it would go right back."[4] The concept of the body as a permanent condition may help explain why the ideal is closer to the reality in Central American and Caribbean countries—there is only so much manipulating that a woman believes she can do, so in striving for her ideal, factors such as owning the right accessories to flatter her shape become just as important as her body itself.

"Jamaicans tend to think of their bodies as relatively unchangeable," agrees Ferguson. "We are born with a certain something that we must do our best with. I myself believe this. You can tone up your muscles a bit and lose or gain a bit of weight here and there, but your basic shape will always return to its natural state."

"Never leave yourself" is a popular expression among teens and young women in Belize, where numerous beauty pageants are held every year and one out of every two high school–age girls claimed to either be participating in a pageant or hopeful of trying out for one.

"The ethnopsychology of this expression, which is deeply rooted in cultural beliefs about the self, serves as a form of self-protection," explains Anderson-Fye. "It is derived from a sense of cultural pride, but the result is to emotionally and physically protect these girls from external influences." The expression is used in conversations beyond body image—girls will fall back on it as an explanation as to why they won't have sex with a persistent boyfriend, why they dress a certain way, or even why they over-slept before school.

Though the phrase is native to Belize, it is echoed by the attitudes of Jamaicans, a culture known for genuine and candid dialogue. ("We say what we mean, even at the risk of insulting the other person," one woman told me.) In such an environment, losing weight for the sake of anyone but yourself is unusual—and losing it for yourself seems foolish, given that curves are highly prized.

The Right Ratio

As the Greeks understood long ago, a beautiful body is quantified not by absolute numbers, but relative ones—proportions that remain constant while individual height and weight may vary. In Jamaica, proper proportion is king. Like the Coca-Cola bottle, which comes in 10-ounce, 12-ounce, and 16-ounce versions, the perfect woman's body in Jamaica may come in small, medium, or large, so long as the dimensions stay true. The bottom should be bigger than the top, and both should be bigger than the middle. "With this ideal," says Anderson-Fye, "it doesn't matter if three women are the same height and one weighs 110, another 140, and the other 170. It's about proportion."

The only body type that does not get respect is a skinny one. "In Jamaica, it has always been better to be 10 pounds overweight than 10 pounds underweight," says Ferguson. In fact, Ferguson's research with psychologist Phebe Cramer, PhD, suggests that this preference starts at a young age:[5] When shown images of other children ranging in size from underweight to obese, Jamaican girls ages 6 to 9 demonstrated significantly less bias against heavier people than their

American counterparts, and in some cases showed favorable bias toward plumpness.

While the ideal holds true across the country, there are gradations: Rural Jamaicans have more prominent curves (though they are by no means obese) than urban women, who tend to fall into one of two categories. Either they are smaller, or they have "lost their curves," as the locals put it, becoming medically obese, which is no longer considered attractive. ("Roundness," as one local woman told me, "means she has forgotten to care for her shape.")

Of course, as with every culture's body ideal, there are some women who come up short—or fall flat, in the case of Jamaica's obsession with curves. But rather than turn to plastic surgery, Jamaicans tend to favor other means of noninvasive enhancement, such as the clever use of clothing and accessories. Shoulder pads, padded bras, a bare midriff, and a bustled skirt are all perfectly acceptable devices used to give the illusion of the perfect body. In the dance halls, flesh is pushed and squeezed into impossibly tiny tops, and jeans cut to accentuate a woman's hips and rear are de rigueur.

For those who feel fashion alone cannot produce the full-figured body they want, there is a growing selection of products that promise smaller women solutions to their lack of the requisite "bump." In fact, over the past 3 decades, several companies have developed products to cure the undercurved population. One such prescription, sold in pharmacies across the country, was called Anorexal, which promised prepubescent girls the curves they were waiting for. (As the name implies, the product was positioned as the antidote to anorexia—not the clinical illness as we define it, but a broader con-

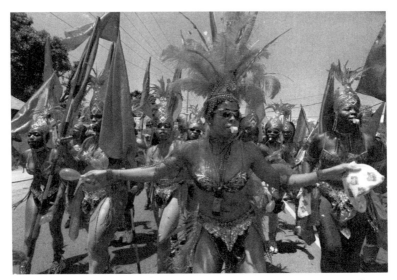

Body Rhythms: Women celebrate Jamaica Carnival 2002 by dancing in the streets in Kingston.

cept derived from the Greek word, which means "loss of a desire for food.") After medical inquiry and heated debate, Anorexal was deemed unsafe and pulled from shelves in the mid-1980s. In its place, pharmacies began to stock Peritol, an antihistamine that purports to enhance the appetite.

While it's true that Jamaican women don't want to change their bodies *too* much, taking supplements that promise to enhance their curves is seen as part of a healthy regimen. "Jamaicans associate size with health and vitality, and a woman absent curves may also be thought of as lacking in good health," explains Sobo.

Since the late 1990s, another trend has emerged: Doctors have noted an increase in the number of young women taking livestock hormones (popularly known as the chicken pill) in hopes of developing larger breasts and bottoms. Alarmed by the practice, the medical community has launched a public awareness campaign about the harmful side effects of such hormones. "These pills are extremely dangerous," says Manuel Pena, MD, a member of Jamaica's Pan American Health Organization. "They are not meant for humans, and taking them can have severe health implications including high blood pressure and metabolic problems."

Nevertheless, the trend appears only to be growing, as those lacking the coveted Coca-Cola–bottle shape are seeking a little help from science.

Arianne's Story

Sexy in our country translates into fleshy thighs, a big bottom, and large breasts. I can attest to this because I do have a slightly large bottom, and this is the feature I receive compliments on.

—ARIANNE ANDERSON, 29,
SCHOOLTEACHER, JAMAICA

As a child, I was teased endlessly for being skinny. Most girls had big bottoms and chests by high school, but I was flat as a board. I remember in eighth grade, a song called "Bumpa Bottom" was popular on the charts. My best friend had a very big bottom, and when we'd go out, she would get many compliments on her "bumpa." Me? I was ignored.

Growing up, I never heard my mother discussing anything about her body. And certainly I didn't bring it up.

But I did understand from an early age that my daddy was very fond of her large bottom and fleshy thighs, as he would jokingly draw attention to them.

At 16, I entered Teachers' College, where I became friends with a group of girls who had the ideal Coca-Cola–bottle shape. I still had no curves. One day, I walked into the college nurses' station with a friend and asked to talk with a nurse about a diet that would help me gain weight. At first, she was amused, but then realizing the seriousness of the matter, she advised me to drink at least three glasses of milk a day for moderate weight gain. Of course, I was not interested in moderate, so for several months, I opted to drink well over seven boxes of milk a day! My friend and I set a goal with a particular pair of shorts: We would continue to drink milk until these shorts no longer fit. Gradually, I began to put on weight. I watched my school uniform get tighter and tighter. Finally, success! I had a bottom I could be proud of.

Suddenly, the catcalls started. Boys who had never made advances began to boldly do so. Some of my male friends coined a term for me, A2K, like Y2K except the A stood for ass. My bottom became my trademark, much to the envy of smaller girls.

The bumpa is an extension of the Coca-Cola ideal. The term is still used, but as fewer glass bottles are used (cans are becoming increasingly popular), I wonder if the next generation will recognize the expression. Still, the ideal is the same: broad hips, flatter stomach, big breasts. We don't obsess too much, though, if our stomach is bigger than we'd like. A walk on the local beaches will bring sights of ladies proudly wearing bikinis with their bellies spilling out. Even the fattest woman in Jamaica will choose the clothing that shows the most of her shape. Jamaican women are very confident in this way.

Much of Jamaican youth today is obsessed with the dance-hall culture, which influences everything from what we wear to how we dance, and in general, how we think about ourselves and our bodies. The dance hall does carry some negative connotations—some say it is vulgar, the explicit language and very sexual moves. Instead, many women, myself included, will go uptown to the nightclubs, which are like the dance halls except a little more upscale. For instance, while a girl going to a nightclub may wear a midriff top, her counterpart at the dance hall may wear only a bra!

Not all dancing is sexual in nature, although most of the songs and movements that come from Carnival, like "Dutty Wine," draw attention to the hips and bottom. It is the girl with the largest bottom that usually gets the attention—she is the one men approach to dance with. I can attest to this because I do have a slightly large bottom, and this is the feature that I get complimented on. I consider my curvy hips and large bottom to be my most attractive physical features, and Jamaican men in my age group find extra flesh on the thighs to be sexy.

When I go out dancing, it is only a matter of time before

I feel a man pressing up behind me, "asking" me for a dance. (This is customary—no man makes verbal requests for a dance!) Occasionally I refuse, simply by turning around so he can no longer feel my bottom. But more often we dance together, gyrating our hips to the rhythms of the reggae. I'll dance from midnight until about 3 a.m., when I go home. After that, it starts to get too outrageous.

You can see from our dancing that proportion of a woman's body is of greatest importance. Your waist might not be small, but if you have bigger breasts and a bottom, then it gives the illusion of a smaller middle. My mother commented that women of my generation seem to have bigger curves than her own generation. I know women who have gone to some drastic lengths to get their curves—one friend took the chicken pill to target those certain areas. I watched her become totally transformed. And she is confident now in her body in a way she was not before.

With our African ancestry, we tend to have larger bottoms to begin with. I think we are just working with what we were given. And Jamaican men always want some meat to grab on to. They'll look at European models in magazines and just laugh. Even today, I am cautious about dieting. My biggest fear, after all that work, is losing my behind.

Body Image, Jamaica-Style

Despite their obvious awareness of a body shape ideal and the care Jamaican women put into attaining that look, the Jamaican body ideal actually relieves Jamaican women of many of the body pressures faced by their peers in other cultures. I found my conversations with Jamaican women to be refreshingly upbeat and lacking in any undertones of gender or political tension—a sharp contrast to talks I've had with my American friends on the same topic. The Jamaican women I spoke with were frank and unapologetic about their bodies, regardless of weight.

In 2008, Phyillicia Bishop, a 20-year-old student at Russell Sage College in Troy, New York, and the first member of her Jamaican family born in the United States, participated in a production of the student play *Mirror, Mirror*, which deals with the topic of body image. "In Jamaica, having a shape is nice," she said.

It seems like something we could all learn from—and indeed, in our globalized world, we very well might start to do so.

CHAPTER 7

BEAUTY AND THE BURKA

*And say to the believing women that they should
lower their gaze and guard their modesty; that they
should not display their beauty and ornaments except
what ordinarily appear thereof; that they should
draw their veils over their bosoms. . . .*

—KORAN, 24:30–31

Under the rickety subway tracks and across the street from a
dusty, noisy cement-making plant, the office occupied by
Women for Afghan Women resides in a dilapidated two-story clap-
board house on the outskirts of Flushing, New York. On the first
floor, a Chinese man who speaks no English runs a store selling
wood paneling. Upstairs, through two sets of locked doors at the end
of a long, dimly lit hallway, I encounter a small piece of paper taped
to the wall that marks the entrance for the nonprofit group's headquarters. It is here that support and counseling are provided for the
approximately 10,000 Afghan immigrants living in the New York
City metropolitan area.

The interior of the Women for Afghan Women's workspace is not much more polished than its exterior. Bare walls and faded charcoal-gray carpets greet me as I step inside. Against one wall, a wooden tabletop is covered with plastic cups and 2-liter soda bottles—leftovers, I learn, from an Afghan New Year's party the previous week.

I am met by Tahera Shairzay, the advocacy program manager for the organization. Dressed in a chocolate-colored zip-up sweater and black slacks, Shairzay wears no head covering, and the gold square nuggets in both of her ears stand out in elegant contrast to her dismal surroundings. "It's temporary," she tells me, indicating that the organization hopes to move to a more central location to better serve their community.

That community is a group of mostly foreign-born men and women earning an average household income of $25,000 a year. Some have emigrated by choice, but most are here because life in Afghanistan, as we well know, has been nearly unbearable for the better part of 25 years.

In 1919, Afghanistan declared its independence from the British government. In the decades that followed, the country found itself increasingly a pawn in international tensions, culminating in the Cold War between the United States and Russia. Because of Afghanistan's proximity to Russia, India, Pakistan, and Iran, Moscow immediately recognized it as a strategic stronghold. America was focused on the country's refusal to sign the Baghdad Pact, a treaty between Iran, Iraq, Turkey, and Pakistan aimed at stabilizing the region. As the United States withdrew its financial support for Afghanistan, the Russians stepped right in, offering technology, weaponry, and financial security to the Afghan monarchy. Quietly, they also offered information on Marxism and labor organization to its people. Social unrest began to build.

"I left my home in Kabul in 1970, to attend American University in Beirut," Shairzay tells me as we sit together in her office. "You had a sense of the Russian influence then, but it was not so bad yet."

In 1973, Afghanistan's leader, King Zahir Shah, was overthrown by a pro-Marxist Afghan regime. Though the new government did not intend to follow Moscow into the arms of full Communism, the door had been opened. Reforms imposed by the Moscow-backed government led to protests and rebellion.

"I returned in 1975 to teach English at the colleges in Afghanistan, then I got engaged and my husband was an engineer who had a job in Saudi Arabia," Shairzay remembers. "So we traveled to Saudi Arabia, where I continued to teach. Our goal was to save enough money to go home and buy a small house in Afghanistan to raise our family. We worked and saved, and our parents found us a home. Two weeks before I was supposed to return to Afghanistan, my parents sent me a telegram. 'Don't come,' they said. 'And don't send us any more money. Things are getting really bad.'" Shairzay remained in Saudi Arabia and watched from afar as her family's world fell apart.

In 1979, the Soviets invaded the country. "There was a strike by the students at Afghanistan's universities, protesting the Russian occupation," she tells me. "My youngest brother was in his final year of college, studying to be an engineer. During the protests, the Russian soldiers started shooting. He was hit by a bullet and went down. When the soldiers got to him, they found anticommunist pamphlets in his pocket. They took him away." Shairzay's father and other brother went looking for him. "They searched every hospital, jail, buildings they knew were pro-Russia. Nothing. But when the soldiers learned who they were, they threw them in jail too." Eventually, Shairzay's father and other brother were released. But her youngest sibling has never been found.

The Taliban seized power from the mujahideen in 1995. At first, many Afghans welcomed what they believed would be a return to order and peace. But in a matter of months, the Taliban began installing such policies as the mandatory wearing of the burka, a complete body and head covering for women; forbidding women to appear in public without a male family member; banning girls from public schools; and then forbidding women to appear in public at all. Though men, too, were forced to follow a strict set of rules, the harshest policies seemed to pertain to women, who had experienced relative freedom and equality under the monarchy in the prewar years.

In fact, some of the women I interviewed recalled wearing provocatively short skirts and Western-style tops in their youth during the 1960s—one woman recalled her mother carefully following the fashions of Western movie stars and incorporating certain looks into her own wardrobe. In general, the fashion was more modest, more conservative in deference to the Islamic tradition. Head scarves were not mandatory, but most women observed some sort of public covering. Burkas were available by choice—and not many young women chose to wear them. Now, suddenly, nothing was by choice, and women found their worlds being determined by a small, powerful group of men.

The Burka and Body Image

This is the backdrop for the question I posed to more than a dozen Afghan women of all ages and economic backgrounds. Many of them now live in the United States, some with hopes of returning home, others with a cynical perspective on what will become of their beloved homeland. I wanted to know: How does the enforced wearing of a burka impact the way women see themselves and their bodies? How do ideas about body and beauty become obscured and altered behind a veil of secrecy?

The ideal body is not something Afghani women frequently discuss. Again and again I am told, with looks ranging from bewilderment to amusement, that there is not the same fixation on body shape within the Afghan culture as there is in the United States.

"We do not think of our bodies as you do," one 40-year-old woman said gently. "We talk about looking good, like a whole presentation, but we do not focus on this body part or that body part. We put together a good package."

So what does an ideal package include? Universally, it includes long black hair, fair skin, and round bodies. *Chubby* is the word used most frequently to describe Afghan women's bodies, and chubby is indeed a good thing to be. "All men like their wives to be chubby," a 79-year-old grandmother of six tells me. "Skinny women will never marry."

At the office of Women for Afghan Women, I ask Shairzay about the Afghan woman's concept of beauty and the ideal body. How is it determined? She, too, is vague in her response, and I have the feeling that she is humoring me, this American reporter who cannot grasp the idea of a culture in which body shape is not a primary fixation among women.

"Unemployment in Afghanistan is so high," she tells me. "And the cost of living in the city, which is the only place you will find work, is also high. Your average family makes $100 or $150 a month. That's with both parents working, and the children working. Afghan families are big—five children is common. Rent for a home in Kabul is $150 to $300 a month. So most people can't afford to live in the city; they live in the ruined buildings on the outskirts of it." With no running water or electricity, life is hard and physically exhausting. An obesity epidemic doesn't seem like much of a threat. As with other countries fighting war and famine, thinness (which is common) is far from an ideal.

"I can remember when I was a girl, and it was summertime and hot and I was running around our house in a sleeveless dress," says Shairzay. "I was extremely thin. My grandmother took one look at me and yelled, 'Tahera, you go put on a shirt to cover your arms! People will say we don't have enough money to feed you!'"

So what, I ask again, would a young Afghan woman say a beautiful body looks like? Shairzay smiles. "You know," she says, avoiding my question, "beautiful women are appreciated all over the world. Gyms, makeup, clothes—these are all things that cost money. Access to them shows that you belong to an economic group very few Afghans can afford to be part of. But beauty you can possess without any of these things." She goes on to remind me that the average Afghan woman rises at sunup, cleans, cooks, fetches water, bathes her children, dresses her children, perhaps leaves for her own job, returns home at sundown, and gets ready to repeat the entire cycle once again the following morning. "Afghan women," she confirms, "have little time to worry about a perfect body shape. But do they like to look good? Of course! This is a universal desire."

Rephrasing the question, I inquire once more what women think of when they think about "looking good." It is hard to get a concise answer. Shairzay describes elaborate fabrics that women buy to sew clothes for special events, as purchasing ready-made clothing in a store is too expensive. She talks about the dirt-cheap makeup, in gaudy colors and thick liquids, that is brought across the border from Pakistan, allowing poorer women the opportunity to make themselves up to their hearts' content (although she clearly disapproves of the over-the-top look some choose to sport). But body shape is not at the top of her list, nor even midpack. I press her to describe the female figure itself— what would an ideal naked lady look like?

"Oh," she says shyly. "Well, the men in Afghanistan like a lot of chubby." Chubby? "Yes, very chubby. Your Barbie, she would not go over very well in Afghanistan." She chuckles at her own mental image. "The Afghan woman's body is most beautiful when it is fleshy, not too skinny. Men do not appreciate that when there is not enough food to eat. Men want their woman chubby."

Shairzay uses the description of "chubby" without any of the negativity that follows when a Westerner chooses such a term. It is a body type we sometimes try to couch nicely as "curvy" or "athletic build," but she sees no need to sugarcoat anything, because frankly, fat is not a bad thing in Afghanistan, especially for women of her generation. In fact, chubby doesn't mean curvy at all, it turns out. Chubby means just that—round, soft, fleshy, overweight. This is a good thing to Shairzay; there is no shame to be felt in chubbiness. As I speak with more and more Afghan women, it becomes clear that not only is the ideal female body heavier than the American standard, but the word *chubby* is clearly the preferred terminology used to (at least in translation) express this aesthetic.

Given what we know about size representing good health and financial security, it is not terribly surprising that a skinny body is unappealing in Afghanistan today. But unlike the Jamaican body standard, which is fuller in size but is defined by specific dimensions of proportion, in Afghanistan there doesn't seem to be any certainty as to what the ideal is (even if they can say what it is not). This brings me back to my original question: Does life beneath the burka—in which all aspects of femininity and body shape are shielded from public view—play into an absence of definitive body ideals? Maybe the figure-forgiving burka frees an Afghan woman from worries about her body. Then again, it seems reasonable to wonder whether covering her body so completely the vast majority of the time would make a woman supremely self-conscious when she does reveal her figure and then most commonly to her husband.

Despite the sinister connotations the burka has in America, not all Afghan women I speak with feel that way, particularly of the older generation. "A lot of Afghan women think of the burka as an overcoat," one 50-year-old woman tells me. "It's convenient if you are heading out to do errands and don't want to have to worry about fixing yourself up first."

To Western ears, this sounds improbably, impossibly, naïve. The burka as we know it is a symbol of all things unequal and unjust to the women of Afghanistan. It is the most obvious indicator of a culture where women are subservient and considered the property of men; where 12-year-old girls are married off for a dowry and 14-year-olds are expected to become mothers.

But Afghan women are much less vocal on this matter. This may be partly because they fear repercussions for their comments, but even Afghan women who have emigrated to the United States don't express the sort of anger and contempt that many Americans project onto the burka. In fact, several Afghan women working for international aid organizations in the United States tell me that while they know the politically correct thing to say here is that the burka is a garment of oppression, they actually do not feel this way, hard as that may be for an American woman to believe.

"The burka is misunderstood," Shairzay flatly tells me. "It is not the invention of the Taliban; it has been part of Afghan culture for centuries. When I was growing up, it was a choice—did you want to wear it or not? I did not wear a burka in Afghanistan, but my aunt wore it all the time, every time she left the house. She said she just felt comfortable in it. During the Taliban, it was no longer a choice. That is the difference."

The burka as a symbol of oppression has been challenged by academic scholars as well. Pekka Rantonen, head researcher of a 2005 study[1] conducted by anthropologists from the University of Tampere in Finland, says that "the automatic equation in the West—wearing a burka means a woman's body is unfit for public viewing, and thus women are suffering and discriminated against—does not hold up in Afghanistan." This doesn't mean women are free from suffering, he points out, only that they do not draw a parallel between their social status and this bodily covering. From Rantonen's research, he concludes that many women see the burka as a symbol of their body's importance. Why would you go to such lengths to conceal something if it were only ordinary? "To cloak so completely a woman's body," he says, "may well be seen as a recognition of its extraordinary beauty and value."

Whether or not covering the body elevates its value, an important by-product of this cloaking is a complete absence of racy billboards or scantily dressed women in advertisements in public spaces. You can call it oppression or exhaltation, but the bottom line is that women in a burka-clad culture are shielded from the bombardment of images that make Western women feel as though they have something they must "measure up" to. The pressure to be a particular body shape is not publicly flaunted for them to see thousands of times every day. Not only is there less pressure, there are fewer reminders, period, that one should be thinking about her body from sunup to sundown. Here, perhaps, is another reason Afghan women seem ambivalent about the concept of an "ideal body."

Given the absence of public displays of flesh, one can imagine the outrage in 2007, when a television station in Mazir-e-Sharif, a relatively progressive city in northern Afghanistan, attempted to launch its equivalent of *America's Next Top Model*, using local women as contestants. Though the show's wardrobe revealed almost no skin and included a mix of traditional and Western dress, more than 20 women backed out due to death threats from Afghan conservatives.

In speaking with women who have seen Afghanistan through

times of relative freedom, oppression, and downright terror, it is clear that they, too, have mixed emotions about the burka and its implications for the way they view their bodies.

Shayma's Story

> *We don't have "body image" like you have in America. We just don't think like that.*
>
> —SHAYMA DANESHJO, 47,
> UNICEF REGION OFFICER, NEW YORK CITY

Growing up in Afghanistan, what I remember about my mother was her elegance. She just had a way of presenting herself. My father once said that a beautiful Afghan woman should have long hair, fair skin, and a chubby body. This was my mother—fair and rounder, with straight black hair—and I thought she was beautiful.

I can honestly say I never worried about my body size or shape when I was growing up, partly because I just assumed I would inherit my mother's genes, and partly because worrying about your weight was not how our society was. Being thin was not a desirable quality for a woman. We frequently watched Bollywood movies from India in the '70s, where the women were curvy. Of course, I remember discussions among my girlfriends over who looked the best. But it was always about the way you presented yourself, not about your body shape.

I grew up just before the Taliban. Afghanistan was a

fairly modern society. Girls attended school; women held good jobs; we had nightclubs and restaurants and parties like any other country. My father worked for the government and my mother was a nurse. I attended an all-girls school where we wore uniforms of black dresses with little white cuffs, thick black stockings, and a white scarf to cover our hair. The uniforms were mandatory because this way you could not separate out which girls came from wealthier families or poorer ones. Outside of school, I wore Western-style clothing. Nothing that showed a lot of skin, but modest skirts and tops.

I first began to think about my body around age 12 or 13—the age when you hit puberty and you are considered a woman. I became aware that my shape was changing. In Afghanistan, this is the point at which your mother becomes your best friend. Girls never talk about intimate topics with their fathers—there is too much tension in that relationship for talk about your body. It is your mother who will share with you the secrets of becoming a woman, finding a husband, and everything that comes from that.

Religion has always played a big role in how Afghan women see their bodies, even before the Taliban. You cover your body in deference to your religious beliefs. In the West it is popular to see the burka as a symbol of all that is oppressive and backward about the lives of Afghan women. I think this is a gross misunderstanding. Yes, for some women, it feels restrictive to be hidden inside this garment. But for others, it is culturally comfortable, a feeling of

safety in an unsafe country. The real issue is about choice—
forcing women to wear a burka is different than allowing
women to choose it.

I don't think the burka itself determines the way women
feel about their looks—good or bad—but it changes the focus
from body to beauty. I'll tell you a story. A few years ago I
was back in Afghanistan, and I was in the remotest, most
desolate area of the country, trying to sign people up to
have their photographs taken for identity cards, so they
could vote in the upcoming elections. And one woman in
line, she must have been in her forties, when she came up to
the booth, she refused to let me take a photograph of her. She
was under her burka, and she told me she was not going to
remove it. I asked her what the problem was, and she said,
"My husband didn't say anything about having a photo
taken. I have not dyed my hair or put on my makeup. I cannot let you take a photograph like this." Remember, we're
talking about the wilderness of Afghanistan. No TV, no
Internet, nothing for her to compare her appearance to. And
yet, her face was the one thing that might be exposed in
public, and she had a definite idea about what would make
it more beautiful. So I believe women have an instinctive
idea about beauty.

Despite living in Afghanistan during a time of openness
and modern thinking, I was not prepared for American culture when I arrived here. I was used to seeing my body as a
small piece of a larger package that includes makeup, hair,
and dress. I was amazed how much money and time is spent

selling products to women to make their bodies thinner, their skin more beautiful. American women are convinced they have to follow a very specific regimen to look good— everything is media driven. Eventually, you become one of them—what else can you do? It's hard to imagine Afghan women could ever have the same insecurities about their bodies like the women here, but it's hard to say, because right now, the issues they face are so much more than about how they look. Obsessing of your body size is a luxury that women in my country simply don't have time for.

Working It Out

While the older generation of women seems incapable of finding the words to describe their body ideal (probably, as I'm starting to realize, because they haven't formulated such a standard in quite the same way some other cultures have), the younger generation—who were in their infancy during Taliban years and are still young enough to enjoy some relative freedoms in the current political climate— have, if not a more definite idea of an ideal, then at least a greater interest in the topic and in their own body shape.

Fitness centers are popping up all over Afghanistan, from Kabul to Herat and every major city in between. In fact, the Cooperation for Peace and Unity (CPAU), a nonprofit organization founded in 1996 to promote conflict resolution and negotiation strategies in Afghanistan, has just launched Fighting for Peace, a boxing class (of all things) for Afghan women in Kabul.

It's a fascinating, if somewhat ironic, idea. Exercising the principles of peace through combat? I call the program's director, Kanishka Nawabi, who is based in London, to learn more. He agrees it's an unusual approach to spreading ideas of conflict resolution, but adds, "when every nongovernmental organization in Afghanistan is promoting workshops to teach women how to sew or make crafts to sell, I think it's refreshing to offer them another way to express themselves, another way to feel empowered, and that's what we are trying to do."

The program, which currently enrolls about 20 young women, ages 15 to 26, seems to hold the most appeal for families returning from refugee camps in Iran and Pakistan. These girls did not experience the harshest Taliban rules, he explains, and returning to a society where those who did are somewhat shell-shocked can cause friction. Boxing becomes an outlet for those emotions. I ask him what the women wear when they box.

"They wear Western-style gym clothes," he tells me. "We hold the classes in the old coliseum in Kabul, where the Taliban used to perform public hangings of those who did not abide by their rules. Now, instead, these women are learning to be athletes." But they do, he adds, wear a burka or some kind of complete covering on the journey to and from their classes.

Although most gyms in Afghanistan cater to the wealthy and the international community, some sports programs, such as CPAU's, are free and thus open to women of all economic classes. Nawabi says feedback from the program's participants has been overwhelmingly positive. "They talk about what it has done for their self-esteem on many levels," he says. "Of course, the ability to take care of one's body through exercise is very important. But also, simply signing up for these classes gives women a purpose, a reason for leaving their homes and going out, and then what they are learning—the ability to defend themselves and protect their bodies at a time when attacks against women are again on the rise—this all adds up to a program that women find empowering in more ways than just body confidence."

Of course, participation still requires family consent—even now women cannot make the decision to join without approval of their fathers or husbands. Nawabi does not see the contradiction in that. "It is in the best interest of the women that they have family consent," he explains. "It is dangerous for women to act against the wishes of their family."

Still, he notes, those who have joined the program fast become role models for other girls and young women in their communities. "You see our students in Western gym clothes—some wearing a head scarf, others not—looking strong and proud of their bodies," he says. "People notice them on the streets. Many of the women have started cutting their hair shorter, and wearing pants. I would not say they want to look like a man, but they are presenting their bodies in a very bold way for Afghanistan. It is impossible not to notice this confidence."

In this way, Afghanistan's younger generation is developing a sense of their bodies that their mothers' generation seems to have not. With greater awareness, I suspect, will come more specific body ideals, as I discover when I talk with Razeia Gulam-Rasul, a boisterous, chatty 17-year-old from Kabul, one of five children born to a welder and schoolteacher. She spent several years living in refugee camps in Pakistan during the war. With long, dark hair and a slim figure, Razeia is the captain of her all-girls soccer team, a first in her country. Her athletic pursuits haven't been without their struggles, but she is relentless in her passion for the sport, which, she says, has given her new confidence in her body's abilities.

Razeia's Story

We don't worry about being skinny.

—RAZEIA GULAM-RASUL, 17,
SOCCER PLAYER, KABUL

I did not go to school until I was 13 years old. In Pakistan, I worked to support my family. I made rugs to sell when we stayed in the camps until the war was over. I returned to Afghanistan in 2002. I guess I thought the country would look beautiful, but everything was ruined. The buildings, the houses, they were all destroyed.

My parents sent me to school once we were back. Most girls here get married at age 15 or 16, but my parents told me, "No, you will finish your education first." It's hard because most Afghan schools are only for 4 hours a day, but I go to an international school and it lasts all day long. Afterward, I hurry to get to the soccer field to play. I am our team captain.

I first saw soccer on the television, and it just looked like fun. Now I play all the time. I can't imagine life without soccer. I like the way it makes me feel, I like the way it makes my body strong. On my sister's wedding day, I was all dressed up in my formal clothes and high heels, when a friend of mine came over to see me. She said, "Let's go play some soccer." I had to go! So I went and played in my good clothes, and when I came home my mother was so mad. She said, "What happened to you?" And I told her I couldn't help myself—soccer means everything to me.

A lot of women in Afghanistan do not take care of their bodies. They do not know about good health and about how to eat right. Even the younger generation thinks it is good to be a little bit fat. I don't know why. No one wants to be skinny. Older women are very happy to be fat. My mother used to be fat in this way, but then she had an illness and now she is thinner. Also, it is much more important how you behave if you want to be considered beautiful. Older women will say that a girl is beautiful if she treats other people with respect. We don't have this obsession with our bodies; beauty is the whole person. With girls my age, it is a little different because some of us know it is not good to be too fat. Like the other day my girlfriend said to me, "Razeia, I am worried I look too fat." And I told her no, she was beautiful just the way she was. So I personally don't like to be fat the way a lot of other girls do, but I would never want to be skinny either.

I like the way I am. I like my body, and I like how my body feels when I play soccer. We don't show off our bodies the way you do in the US. For one thing, that would be dan-

*gerous. I don't wear a burka, but I always wear a long coat
down to my knees over my blue jeans. And I cover my head
with a scarf. If you show too much of your body, the boys
will be mean to you. They will call you names and ask you
who you think you are to dress in such a way.*

*In the US, I know people go to gyms. But in Afghanistan,
playing sports is the way you take care of your body. Girls
are not allowed to run in Kabul, except on the sport field. My
female soccer team has received some threats. We went to an
international competition in the US not long ago, and when
we came back, our neighbors threatened my family so much
harm that we had to move. But I won't ever stop playing soccer. This is how I take care of my body and my health.*

The Fear Factor

For every story of hope like Razeia's, there are also stories of set-
backs. Nineteen-year-old track star Mehboba Ahdyar was permitted
to join Afghanistan's four-member Olympic team for the 2008
Games in Beijing. She was the only female athlete representing her
country, and though her finishing times in the 800 and 1,500 meters
were below average, her mere presence spoke volumes about the
country's growing interest in women in sports. In a newspaper interview before the Games, Ahdyar's mother, Moha Jan, said, "We are
scared of the people who have a negative view of my family [for
allowing Mehboba to compete], but this will not stop us from supporting our daughter."

Soon after the Western press caught wind of Ahdyar's training, however, the family began receiving death threats. Ahdyar was followed on several of her training runs, and despite her adherence to the rigid Afghan standards for covering her body by wearing a baggy tracksuit and head scarf to run in 100-degree heat, members of her community vocalized their disapproval. Ahdyar began training at night so that no one could see her. But the threats of harm continued. In July 2008, during a brief stay at an Olympic training camp in Italy, Ahdyar disappeared. Several days later, she resurfaced and announced her withdrawal from the Games and quest for asylum in Europe.

Still, the movement for control over one's body, if not in a political sense then at least in a personal one, continues its forward march. In other regions of the country, the trend of women's physical fitness is slowly catching on. Part of the appeal appears to be that the health clubs provide a safe, women-only environment for friends to meet and socialize. In Herat, a Gold's Gym (no relation to the US franchise) boasts more than 50 female members. Its founder, Elham Pirooz, was the first to open a public fitness facility in the city in 2005. She charges members $4 a month (a fee that still relegates the activity to the financially advantaged) for use of the machines and classes that include bodybuilding and karate. As with many of the more outgoing young women in Afghanistan, Pirooz spent most of her childhood outside of the country, living in Iran during the Soviet occupation and Taliban years. Now that she has returned, she is helping to shape the future of her country.

It is too soon to tell what shape Afghan women's body ideals will take in the future—every week there are more stories of Taliban resurgence and attacks on women who attempt to assert their independence, despite the government's stated belief in greater gender equality. What *is* clear to me, from my conversations with Afghanistan's women, is that in order for the concept of a body ideal to take form, a sense of personal safety is essential. Maintaining and perfecting one's body will always take a backseat to the primary goal of protecting it.

CHAPTER 8

WHEN TECHNOLOGY CAME
TO TOWN

*I think it's fair to say that personal computers have
become the most empowering tool we've ever created.
They're tools of communication, they're tools of
creativity, and they can be shaped by their user.*

—BILL GATES, FOUNDER, MICROSOFT

T ype the words *ideal body* into Yahoo's search engine, and you'll
be rewarded with no fewer than 120,000,000 hits. Among
these results is a site called www.createyouridealbody.com, where
you can find a personal life coach to help you achieve the body you
want (no exercise required!), as well as a site called www.idealbody4u.
com, which provides hypnosis and other mind-altering techniques
to help you think your way thin. The sheer volume of opinions,
images, and information available online is head-spinning. But the
overriding message is clear: Your ideal body is likely smaller than

the one you have, and there is an entire industry devoted to helping you achieve your goal.

With just one click, you also can find out about the top fashion trends in Paris (www.parisfoto.com), discover the most popular places in China to get plastic surgery (www.evercare.com.cn), and check out which teeny bikinis the curvy bodies of Brazilian women are sporting this season (www.bikinisbrazilian.com). While the popularity of these images endures, the novelty has worn off for most Americans. After all, television has been beaming images from faraway lands into our homes for several decades. The Internet simply provides slightly more raw footage—citizen journalism instead of the evening news.

But imagine living in a developing nation where access to television is minimal and access to the Internet is nonexistent. Imagine that international phone calls are prohibitively expensive, and anyway, you don't know anyone outside your immediate community whom you'd ring up even if you could pay for it. Imagine that the whole world as you know it reflects only what's happening on your street, in your neighborhood. Then, imagine waking up one morning to discover that a hotel is being built in your village to house the thousands of tourists who want to enjoy the blissfully good weather of your remote country. As it caters to a clientele of wealthy foreigners, it will offer its guests all of the amenities they would expect in a Western hotel: telephones, televisions, fitness centers. You and the other locals who are hired to work at the hotel can catch glimpses of television shows in the restaurants and bars that you staff and rooms that you clean. For some, it is the first time you will see an American soap opera. You may not understand what is being said, but you do understand that these tall, thin, long-haired women are dressed in expensive clothing and seem to enjoy a glamorous lifestyle. This is America, you think. This is what it means to have money.

Five years later, television sets have become a luxury that some of your more affluent neighbors can afford. Friends crowd into one another's two-room houses on weekday nights to share drinks, swap gossip, and watch one of the Western imports. Your country's fledgling entertainment industry is trying to launch a locally produced show, but it's hard to compete with the big-budget programs beamed in from across the ocean.

A decade more down the road, a new construction industry is booming. Towers are being erected on the unblemished land for cell phone and Internet reception. At first, the Internet seems strange and cold and entirely unappealing—useful for businesspeople on holiday who need to check in with their offices and not much else. But bit by bit, your children and their friends begin to experiment with this new device. *Did you know that you can send a message to someone in another country for free?* they ask each other. The appeal of connecting with peers—anytime you feel like it—is irresistible. And in the course of 20 years, your small country is transformed from an isolated island to a nation fully integrated in a two-way exchange of ideas and information about everything from fashion to politics to pop culture.

What sounds like a textbook tale concocted to illustrate the march toward globalization is, in reality, a thumbnail sketch of life in Fiji over the past 2 decades. When you hear the name Fiji, you probably think of sunshine, sand, and bronzed bodies. And for many years, that image would have been correct; the stereotype of the easygoing islander was a more or less apt description of the island's inhabitants. The landscape was beautiful. The pace was leisurely. And the women—well, the women were worshipped by the men for their undeniably beautiful bodies. But probably not in the way you're thinking.

"In the 1950s, women in Fiji were generally short—maybe 5 feet 3 inches—and by American standards, they were fat," says Anne Becker, MD, a medical anthropologist at Harvard University and head researcher for numerous studies about Fijians and body image. The preference for larger bodies, Becker believes, was driven by the familiar equation of body size and personal wealth. Furthermore, the traditional Fijian style of dance, not dissimilar to native Hawaiian dancing, emphasized movements of the belly and hips, so it would make sense, she says, for the idealized body to accentuate these areas.

In 1989, Becker and her team of researchers visited the fishing villages of Fiji to conduct in-depth research on body image. Becker encountered a culture of women virtually devoid of any concerns about shape and size. It wasn't that they weren't aware of their size relative to other women, she explains, but rather, since a larger size was considered a positive attribute—and most Fijian women tended to be on the heavier side—there was little to stress over. Secondly, even those who expressed a degree of insecurity about their bodies felt no motivation to change the way they looked. "The Fijians' explicit attentiveness to fluctuations in weight and body size is often registered in insults associating weight loss and thinness with social neglect or deprivation and compliments relating a robust form with healthy vigor and social connectedness," she writes. "However, while there seems to be a consensual preference for particular ideal physical attributes in Fiji, there is a striking absence of interest in attaining these as a personal goal."[1]

At the time of Becker's first visit, the average body mass index for Fijian women was 29.8. (In the United States, 30 or above is considered obese.) A full two-thirds of all adults were significantly overweight or obese. The remarkable thing, notes Becker's fellow researcher Eileen Anderson-Fye, PhD, an anthropologist at Case Western Reserve University in Cleveland, is that none of these women had a concept of heaviness as a negative, nor did they perceive themselves to be "big" in the American sense of the word. Instead, most women grossly underestimated their own size and expressed a desire to actually gain more weight. (Becker herself gained almost 20 pounds while doing her research in Fiji—every time she went to someone's home to conduct an interview, they insisted on feeding her, first as an act of hospitality and second as a sign of concern for her slimness.)

Becker's team was the first group of anthropologists to study body image and ideals among Fijian women. Leaving behind a weight-obsessed culture, the American scientists found the Fijians' enthusiasm for large size astounding. "There were definite opinions about the ideal body," notes Anderson-Fye, "just not in the way we'd been conditioned to think about it." Comments about a rotund shape, for both women and men, were regularly integrated into everyday Fijian dialogue. For instance, Becker reported:

"Fijians often greet acquaintances by remarking that they appear *colacola vina*, which literally means 'healthy' but also connotes robust appearance with respect to weight. There are also frequent explicit remarks on the appearance and general shape of others. For example, when favorably impressed, Fijians describe a person as *juba vina* (well formed), which generally refers to a full, though not obese, form."[2]

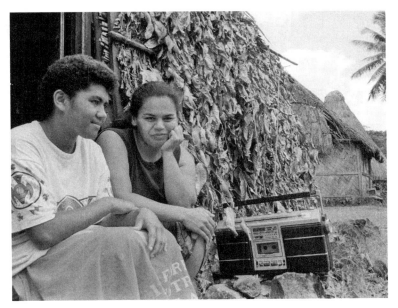

The Way It Was: Fijian women sit outside their homes in Suva, Fiji, in 1997, listening to the radio. Before TV made its way into the homes of everyday Fijians in the mid 1990s, many Pacific islanders relied on the radio for international news and entertainment.

Becker further explained that the ideal female shape, by Fijian standards, was one where a woman looked strong enough to withstand the physical labor required for life in a Fijian fishing village. "One young man . . . said men notice the shape of women before anything else 'because you can see in the shape . . . the ability to work hard,'" she said. A bigger size signaled she'd be better equipped to help with physically demanding jobs; skinny meant she'd watch while he worked.

In 1998, 10 years after Becker's original visit to the island, she returned to the villages of Fiji to see how her subjects—many of whom were young girls when she first visited—had grown. What she found was shocking: "In the span of 1 decade, women and girls went from embracing 'big is beautiful' to an eating disorder rate of 15 percent," Becker says. "There was a complete reversal of cultural ideals for women's body size."

It would be reasonable to think that such a dramatic shift in ideals must have been prompted by an equally intense political or social event—some sort of cultural revolution. But actually, the first cases of eating disorders in the small villages where Becker conducted her research can be traced to a seemingly much more benign occurrence. In the fall of 1995, "TV 'came' to the island's fishing villages," says Becker. "One or two resorts had access before, but the country's new infrastructure [in terms of the installation of electrical and television cables] meant suddenly, for the first time, the average Fijian had the ability to access a television set."

The complete absence of eating disorders or awareness thereof prior to this point is supported by the fact that locals had no term for the behavior of self-starvation. Calling a woman thin was as offensive, in our context, as calling someone "fatso." Within 18 months of the mass distribution of television into everyday people's homes, doctors documented the first known case of anorexia on the island: the patient was a 15-year-old girl.

"The widespread viewing of television was the Fijians' first chance to intensely study the behaviors and values of the Western world," Becker notes. "And what the soap operas and sitcoms conveyed was that a successful, desirable woman was always dressed to kill and always, *always* skinny."

Sharon's Story

There was no television on the island when I grew up. My biggest influence was Bollywood—Indian films with beautiful, curvaceous actresses.

—SHARON BHAGWAN ROLLS, 42, DIRECTOR OF A NONPROFIT IN SUVA, FIJI

TV came to most of the island in the early to mid-1990s. Before that, it was cinema that gave us our entertainment, usually Bollywood films where voluptuous actresses wore skimpy dresses. I'd go with my family every 2 weeks or so; it was a big event. In the late '70s and early '80s, I remember seeing the James Bond movies, too, but I never wanted to look like a Bond girl.

Along with the introduction of TV in Fiji have come changes in people's lifestyles. It used to be you would come home and everyone would gather around and talk about the day over dinner. Now, mealtime centers on grabbing food and sitting in front of the television. In urban areas like where I live in Suva, kids are addicted to the Internet. I have a 16-year-old daughter and 19-year-old son, and I have to monitor how much time they spend online. In rural areas, women still do physical work, on plantations, farming, fishing, taking things to sell at market. But it's not like that in the city. So when I talk to my daughter about a "good body," I talk about living a healthy lifestyle. Healthy is the message we need to stress in Fiji—not skinny like the women on TV.

Now, telling someone they've gained weight is definitely a put-down in Fiji. There are older women I know—friends and relatives—who still think of me like I am 16 years old. And when they see me, they'll happily say, "Oh, you've put on weight!" The last time someone said that to me, I got upset. Would my size have mattered back 30 years ago? Probably not. Times have changed.

It's the Media's Fault

For decades in the United States, psychologists have been researching the theory that the images of ultrathin women in the media negatively impact women's body confidence. Several studies show that women or girls who are exposed to these images experience varying degrees of unhappiness with their bodies and a desire to lose weight. Research also suggests that when women compare themselves to these "perfect bodies," the emphasis is generally upward, not downward—in other words, rather then being pleased with their similarities to these bodies, they tend to focus only on the qualities they don't have.[3] In general, such comparisons result in women feeling less attractive than they did prior to viewing these images. In fact, a 2006 study found that women who read fashion magazines while eating lunch or dinner actually stop eating their meals, feeling subconscious pressure to trim inches from their own waistlines.[4]

But the impact of these images seems to be further heightened when technology is thrown into the mix—that is, when the women being held up for comparison appear on popular television shows such as *Friends* or *Sex and the City* or when the images are available via the Internet. Linda Jackson, PhD, a professor of psychology at Michigan State University in East Lansing who specializes in research on gender and technology, explains, "TV and movies present walking, talking, emoting images of women. Compare this to the still, inanimate images of women you see in magazines, and it's clear that women you can observe *doing* things are much more captivating and engaging to the viewer." We like Jennifer Aniston's character on *Friends*; we are awestruck by sexy, powerful Angelina Jolie gliding down the red carpet with her beautiful family in tow. They are enviable; we want to be like them in a way that few of us would feel toward a *Vogue* model. We are captivated by the personalities of these women we see on television or the big screen. We want to look like them, and feel like failures when we discover that we cannot.

If such images have a significant impact on the self-perception of women in the United States, who are aware and vocally critical of the marketing machine behind them, it's easy to see how women who are viewing them for the first time—and with no context—may find them intimidating. And theoretically, in a relatively poor country where largeness is preferred, such images might be downright off-putting. After all, a comprehensive study published in the 2007 issue of *Epidemiologic Review*, which compiled 333 studies on body image conducted over 16 years from a wide range of countries, concluded that "the overall pattern of results . . . was of an increasing proportion of positive associations [with obesity] and a decreasing proportion of negative associations [with obesity] as one moved from countries with high levels of socioeconomic development to countries with medium and low levels of development. . . . Negative associations for women in highly developed countries were most common with education and occupation."[5]

And yet today's young Fijians do not comply with this finding. Instead, as Becker discovered, televised images of skinny Western women appear to have directly contributed to a rise in eating disorders, an increase in body dissatisfaction, and a new emphasis on weight loss. Given these changes in behavior, it's only logical to say that television—or at least, the images it projects—caused a paradigm shift in Fijian body ideals at an alarmingly speedy rate.

In researching this cultural about-face, I was struck by the apparent lack of resistance to the introduction of a new ideal. After all, Jamaica and South Africa are both economically challenged countries with access to American television shows and fashion magazines. But there the Western body ideal, though not invisible, is kept in check by an overwhelming majority who prefer the traditional body shape—rounder in South Africa, curvier in Jamaica. The stronger influences of health and lifestyle ensure that traditional body preferences dominate.

Which leads to a question, then: What are the driving factors shaping Fiji's culture in the late 20th and early 21st century? Why do these variables make it so easy to assimilate the Western body ideal into the Fijian psyche? The answer, most likely, lies in the fastest-growing force behind the South Pacific's economy: American tourist dollars. According to a 2007 report from the region's marketing and development organization, tourism in the year 2000 brought about 1 billion US dollars into the economy.[6] Four years later, the number grew to $1.5 billion. The organization projects that by 2010, tourist dollars will account for $2 billion fed into the local economies of the South Pacific islands.[7] By comparison, the entire gross domestic product of Fiji in 2007 was $2.43 billion. Meanwhile, the Fiji High Commission on Tourism reported that tourism is Fiji's fastest-growing industry in terms of job creation and foreign exchange earnings. By the end of 2009, the government expects that one in every four jobs in the country will be in the travel and tourism business.[8] Long-term projections are that one in every 3.6 Fijians will work in the industry by 2019. As an indication of the economic importance of tourism, when political unrest in 2007 caused tourists to rethink a Fiji vacation, the local economy shrank by 4 percent.

Who are the visitors to Fiji, introducing the locals to new ideas, ideals, and aesthetic choices? The country receives tourists from across the globe, but the vast majority are white and/or Western. Nearby Australia accounts for one-third of all foreign visitors, followed by New Zealand, the United States, and the United Kingdom. (US numbers are rapidly rising, since major airlines began offering direct flights from Los Angeles in 2004.)

What all this means is that, for starters, the largely agricultural country has quickly become dependent on pleasing the preferences of foreigners. And in ways South Africa and Jamaica don't experience, tiny Fiji is saturated with the presence of their wealthy guests. Its population of 932,000 plays host to more than 500,000 tourists annually, compared to, say, the 48.8 million South Africans who hosted about 9 million foreign visitors in 2007 (a 5.5:1 ratio, versus Fiji's 2:1). So, not only is the US dollar via the tourist industry essential, but the average Fijian is much more likely to have daily contact with the people spending those dollars. Such proximity to wealth on the part of the poor locals, I'd argue, makes Western ideas about beauty and bodily perfection that much more a part of their everyday reality.

One might also argue that the incentive for tourists to come to Fiji is different than, say, for the American tourist in Jamaica, where the "vacation experience" is marketed as a chance to let it all hang out in a fun-loving, reggae-listening, rum-drinking, party-dancing culture. You go to Jamaica to sample the *Jamaican* life. You go to Fiji, on the other hand, for the tranquil honeymoon, the chance to be pampered and attended to, the possibility of having the very best of Western luxuries transported to the setting of an island paradise.

Television sets became standard fixtures in Fijian homes at the same time that the Fijian government began to invest millions into a service industry that catered to a group of people who very much resembled the ones on TV. As more and more foreign tourists came to the island, the fantasy playing out on Fijians' television screens began to reflect the reality of the faces (and bodies) on their island. The Western aesthetic, reinforced by its financial connotations, became that much more difficult to resist.

Abby's Story

Young women in Fiji want to go the extra mile to look like the women on TV. These images set the current standards for beauty.

—ABBY YOUNG, 23, TELEVISION PRODUCER, FIJI

I have an interesting perspective on the ideal woman's body because I was born in Suva, Fiji; spent my teenage years in American Samoa; and now live in Fiji again as an adult.

When I lived in Samoa, I visited my family in Fiji every summer. Like many people in the South Pacific, my heritage is mixed. I am part Tongan-Chinese-Fijian-Indian-Samoan and Rotuman. I have the best of all worlds, I guess.

In Fiji, women my age form a standard for their appearance based on the international TV shows that have recently been introduced, and the music videos and reality shows we get from the US. Maybe this is why here, as in the US, "weight watching" is of high interest to the women. Young women exercise and play sports, especially netball. I used to go to the gym every day, but my job at the TV station makes it difficult. Instead, I joined my company's soccer team. A lot of women here prefer sports to the gym.

Like most women my age, I look to TV for ideas about beauty. I work as a presenter for our local TV music show and as a producer for a show about Fiji's Hibiscus Festival (which has a beauty pageant). I've brought a lot of American fashions with me from Samoa to wear on these programs. I started watching TV when I was about 5—American and some British imports. I don't remember there being any local shows. Today we get Extra *and* Project Runway *and MTV, shows that have a big impact on the styles of teens and women my age. I even notice some locals fronting accents because Westerners from overseas are viewed as popular and cool.*

Much has changed in Fiji in recent years as far as appearance goes. We have transitioned from traditional images of fuller-bodied women to more Western ideas about beauty. For women of my grandmother's generation, a rounder figure was definitely preferred. But in the '90s there was a shift to a thinner body.

Where are we headed in Fiji? I don't see any backlash to Western influence happening here. I believe as trends evolve through the media—on TV and the Internet—the Western influence will only grow stronger. I don't think it's a bad thing. The women here know they are beautiful in their own way. I truly don't know of any girls with eating disorders. I think a Western influence adds something extra.

A New Twist on Technology

If television—and its mostly Western programming—has served as a one-way exchange of cultural information, the introduction of the Internet has had an entirely different effect. Suddenly, young women aren't exposed solely to Western bodies and attitudes. Instead, Web sites such as Friendster and Facebook, highly popular with teens in the States, have opened brand-new lines of communication for young people in Fiji—and dozens of other wired countries across the globe. Want to know what's cool in China? Who's wearing what in Russia? These social networking sites for teens offer instant access to "friends" around the world. What are other girls talking about, or dressing like? The answers are instantaneous. Here, in communities around the world, the global exchange of information is increasing, and it's virtually unstoppable among users who enthusiastically post a steady flow of e-mails and photos for others to read, view, and comment on. Home pages are tickets to new—or perhaps simply more honest—identities, allowing their creators to write anything they want about themselves.

And through video sites such as YouTube, young women from around the world can also view the looks, body types, and fashion styles of their international peers. There they can see real girls and women, not models, with real bodies and a sense of street fashion trends. But beyond the novelty of having a "friend" in Tokyo or Sydney, the Internet provides a vehicle through which its users can affirm their own body image and get a glimpse of what other girls around the world think is "ideal"—or simply "normal."

And so, while researchers such as Linda Ricciardelli, PhD, have found that the influence of television has prompted the younger generation of Fijian women to express virtually the same concerns about weight gain as their Western counterparts, concluding that "the Western ideals are the ones being promoted by the media—which is largely run by Western companies in countries like Fiji,"[9] the Internet may prove to soften that desire. Broadening Fiji's exposure to Western ideals temporarily flattened body image in this part of the globe in the early 21st century. But an even greater expansion of global information exchange has provided the platform for a broader worldview—one that will perhaps, with time, allow Fiji's curvier landscape to reemerge.

CHAPTER 9

A GENERATIONAL REVOLT

My son is my son till he gets him a wife, but my
daughter's my daughter all the days of her life.

—JAPANESE PROVERB

"I can tell a Japanese woman by looking at her feet," says Paco Underhill, CEO of Envirosell, one of the leading market research companies in the United States, and author of the bestseller *Why We Buy*, a book on the science of shopping. Envirosell has offices in 26 countries, including Tokyo, Sao Paulo, Moscow, and Milan, and works with global-reaching clients, from McDonald's to Bulgari. As we sit in his office in Manhattan's Flatiron neighborhood, Underhill explains the critical ways in which companies that market their products internationally must distinguish among their female clientele.

This knowledge is crucial because what sells in Kyoto does not necessarily correlate to what sells in Shanghai, and what's hot on Madison Avenue most certainly does not promise the same brisk sales in Tokyo's high-end Ginza shopping district.

"More specifically," Underhill continues, "by the way she walks.

One of the biggest mistakes is to assume you can lump all Asian cultures into the same market. Korean women, for instance, walk with a manly stride—big steps, perhaps left over from the way they used to have to push their big skirts out of the way as they moved. Japanese women, though, tend to take small steps, and their feet point inwards." This, Underhill speculates, may be a remnant from centuries of fashion that dressed women in tightly wound kimonos, making any sort of grand movement impossible and constricting a woman's strides to minimal dimensions.

What do pigeoned toes have to do with body ideals? It's a bit of a circuitous route—or columnar, to be more exact. "The Japanese basis for ideas about feminine beauty and the body begins with the kimono," says Underhill.

From an American point of view, it's difficult to imagine ideals about the perfect body being dictated by a single garment of clothing. In our culture today, blue jeans perhaps come the closest to determining a desirable body shape (especially given the "skinny jean" phenomenon), but even these are available in different shapes and sizes tailored to individual body types. The kimono, on the other hand, offers little variance in shape and cut (though patterns and colors change). Given its omnipresence among the female population for several centuries, its importance as a status symbol, indicator of personal taste, dictator of physical aesthetics, and guideline for body shape cannot be overstated. Takie Lebra, PhD, a scholar in Japanese cultural anthropology who specializes in such topics as gender roles and social organization, concurs.

"Traditional Japanese notions of the desirable female body shape do have a lot to do with the kimono," she says. "The idea is that the body should not be displayed, but rather should be protected and only strategically revealed inside this gorgeous robe. In fact, women wore a *haori* coat over the kimono, especially for more formal occasions, to further prevent displaying their body shape."

At the root of this conservative display of the body lies a set of beliefs about beauty that are uniquely Japanese. For centuries, Japanese beauty has been defined by a philosophy of perfect harmony between mind and body. Unlike Western philosophy, in which the two are treated as separate entities to be nurtured in different ways, in Japan, thought and action, or the intellectual and the physical, are viewed as one. As such, attributes like modesty, discipline, simplicity, and structure also define the Japanese aesthetics for physical beauty, and many traditional art forms, from painting to flower arranging to fashion, exemplify this aesthetic standard. The kimono, with its clean, precise lines, was considered ideal—and by association, the body that fit the kimono was aspired to.

So while the sophisticated ladies of Europe's ballrooms were exposing no small amount of décolletage in their plunging gowns in the 18th century, the women of Japan's high society were baring no more than an Adam's apple in the company of men. Any curves were tightly bound in the kimono. In fact, some literature suggests that women padded their midsections underneath the garment to further flatten their surface. The *obi*, a wide sash worn around the waist, also served to fill out a woman's midsection to continue the desired tubular, linear effect created by the kimono.

Lebra's description echoes the thinking of anthropologist and East Asian scholar Laura Miller, PhD, former president of the American Anthropological Association, who explains the traditional Japanese body ideal as one based on the shape of a rolling pin. "The kimono gives the female form a columnar look that de-emphasizes the breasts and waist and draws attention to the neck, hips, and ankles," she writes in *Beauty Up*, a critical look at the booming cosmetic industry in Japan.[1]

As in any other culture, beauty trends in Japan have come and gone over the centuries (the darkened-tooth preference and practices in the 10th century, when white teeth were considered remarkably unattractive, is one example). But certain physical preferences have remained fairly constant. Smooth, lustrous skin, for example, has always been considered beautiful in Japan, as have, until recently, small, delicate lips. And the nape of the neck, says Miller, has been a focal point of eroticism and sexuality in Japan for more than 2 centuries, owing largely to the fact that it is one of the few areas of flesh actually exposed by the kimono. Even as Western attire has become the norm in modern culture, the nape of a woman's neck still places among the top five erogenous zones in surveys of Japanese men.[2]

Breasts, on the other hand, barely made a blip in Japanese erotica or popular magazines; as recently as the early 1980s, racy, cleavage-bearing photos usually featured foreign women. In fact, throughout Japanese literature, it is difficult to find erotic references to women's breasts.[3] Anthropologists attribute this to the fact that the female breast in Japanese culture is first and foremost associated with motherhood. Breasts are referenced, for instance, in nursery rhymes and bedtime songs. Anthropologist Lebra explains it this way: "In Japan, women's breasts have been adored more as a symbol of maternal nurturance than of sex."[4] Indeed, ample-size breasts were an embarrassment to many Japanese women. As Miller notes, "A derogatory term for women whose large breasts alter the desired pillar shape [of the kimono] is 'pigeon chest' or *hatomune desshiri*."[5] That there is a term for this at all is unusual: Unlike the vagina, which, according to one compendium, has no fewer than 260 slang terms in Japanese, breasts are allotted a measly six.[6]

This apparent lack of interest in breasts is notable, as most cultures—no matter how unique or opposite their body ideals— tend to hold a sexualized view of these parts of the female body. But breasts create curves, and curves disrupt the linear aesthetic that was the Japanese body ideal for centuries. Even now, almost a century past the kimono's popular wear in everyday life, it is still used as a reference point for the perfect female figure.

Kyoko Matsuda, a slender 37-year-old born and raised in Tokyo, would appear by American standards to fit the Japanese ideal. She is about 5 feet 6 inches with silky black hair that falls below her shoulders. Walking across the room of a café, she cuts a slender, delicate silhouette. But Kyoko is less than pleased with her body. "I will never forget, as a young girl, being sized up by one of my relatives and told, 'You do not have a kimono body.' This was said not as a compliment!"

Yumiko's Story

I still remember women wrapping towels around their chests to flatten themselves in their kimonos.

—YUMIKO ADACHI, 57, BUSINESS OWNER, TOKYO

I was born and raised in Tokyo. I divorced when I was 34, and have no children. Growing up, I rarely thought about my body size or shape; for my generation, part of the post-war baby boom, the biggest concern was good health.

I started to think about my body shape and my appearance in my early forties, when I began working out at a health club. My friends from the gym gave me advice. Of course, when Japanese women discuss their bodies, it is rarely about what they like. I never talk with my girlfriends about the good things, only to share complaints.

My feelings about my body are mixed. I'm happy with my firm legs, but I'd like to change some other parts. I don't like my loose waistline, flat buttocks, and flabby upper arms, and I'd like to lose about 8 pounds. I am 5 feet 3 inches and weigh 117 pounds. I think it's average for my age. But since entering my fifties, I'm getting fatter. I no longer fit the Japanese model for an ideal body.

There are certainly aspects of what we find beautiful that share common ground with Western ideas about body and beauty. Japanese women have been attracted to Western women's body shapes all through the ages, but instead of extreme height and super curves, the ideal body for Japanese women of my generation was moderate height, flat, sharp, narrow, and firm. Of course, as my generation gets older, full-time housewives become less and less concerned with what their body looks like. But women with a job are still conscious about their appearance and what other people think of them. I'm very conscious about my body size.

The kimono body type is relevant to our current ideals, but Japanese women's body shapes have changed with the times. We've adopted Western foods and lifestyles, and fitting into a kimono would prove to be a challenge to many today!

Of course, in addition to adopting Western women's lifestyles, we've taken on some of their sense of style and body ideals as well. Many young women now dye their hair, something that began about 20 years ago. But whereas for American women the ideal body is about looking sexy, Japanese women focus more on how to look beautiful. This is an important distinction because for us, the idea of physical beauty cannot be separated from mental stability, strength, and balance. Japanese culture still considers the whole person in evaluating something like beauty. To have a well-balanced diet, moderate exercise, satisfying work, and good relationships with family, friends, and a partner— these are all taken into consideration as part of what makes a woman "beautiful" in Japan.

Men's opinion about the "perfect body" for women is often different from our own. But women don't listen to men! In truth, I'm not sure Japanese husbands care whether their wives are gaining weight or losing weight. They do not pay attention to subtle changes in the body the way women do.

New Looks for New Times

Today on the streets of Tokyo, advertisements for push-up bras, breast augmentation, and other pseudoscientific means of developing bigger, perkier chests seem to be proliferating. "You see everywhere in Tokyo now ads for products that make you look taller, slimmer, bigger-chested," says Kyoko Matsuda. "Women in Japan are very, very interested in looking good." Are Western ideals creeping into a culture previously impervious to such an aesthetic?

It's not that simple. In the 1980s, Japanese fashion became notable for an odd, somewhat disturbing trend: Grown women— educated, career-minded twentysomethings—developed a sudden affection for knee socks, plaid skirts, and Hello Kitty purses. Seemingly overnight, stores sold tens of millions of dollars worth of Hello Kitty merchandise. Covers of popular fashion magazines like *Denjeki Layers* and *Cosmode* featured women wearing their hair in pigtails. Japanese porn shops peddled videos of women looking so childlike it bordered on pedophilia. To foreigners, it was nearly comical to see adult women trying to look like 12-year-olds in girls-school uniforms. But the trend tapped into an aspect of physical idealization in Japan (shared by many other cultures): the innocent virgin. A flat-chested, schoolgirlish appearance represented the proverbial unplucked rose—naive, delicate, and pure. "Japanese men have always desired 'cute' girls instead of women," Kyoko tells me.

But this was the eighties, and another trend was on the rise along with the fashion explosion of "cute." During this decade, there was a 50 percent increase in women joining the workforce. As high-pressure jobs and 12-hour workdays became the norm for young women, the image of banker Soo in her blue pinstripe suit was juxtaposed uncomfortably next to the model toting her pink Hello Kitty shoulder bag on the billboards across Tokyo. It seemed something would have to give: A 35-year-old vice president of a bank was unlikely to don knee-high socks and pigtails on the weekends. As Japan entered the last decade of the 20th century, it was clear that the new model for young Japanese women was strong, smart, and in control. It was time her clothing—and the body wearing it—caught up with her brain.

As Yumiko Adachi pointed out when I interviewed her, when it comes to Japanese perceptions of beauty, the mental and physical are strongly intertwined. (It is not by accident that Japanese designer Kihachiro Onitsuka created an athletic footwear company in 1977 called ASICS—an acronym for *Anima Sana in Corpore Sano*, which translates as "strong mind, strong body.") So as strong, educated, independent-minded women began to enter the workforce en masse, they demanded—and could afford—bodies that reflected their minds.

A Culture of Work Meets "Working Out"

In the 1980s, most young Japanese women lived at home with their parents while pursuing postcollege careers (as this is customary in their culture, many young women still do so today). Imagine, no rent or mortgage bills to pay! What else to do but spend the majority of their paychecks on the latest trends in fashion and beauty?

"With a disposable income and untethered to children and a husband, the unmarried young woman had the freedom to sample a variety of activities," writes anthropologist Laura Spielvogel in her book *Working Out in Japan*. It wasn't long before a fledgling fitness industry began to form and rapidly attract female members. In 1980, there were fewer than 100 health clubs in all of Japan. By 2006, there were more than that in Tokyo alone. The popularity of working out can best be understood by what we already know about Japanese culture and the perception that beauty comes from mind and body working in tandem. While aerobics classes and health clubs may be American imports, the concept of fitness—regardless of its Western influence—appears to be strongly reaffirmed by Japanese tradition. "The import and subsequent popularity of aerobics and fitness clubs coincided with the height of the bubble economy, the growth of the service sector, and the emergence of the female-oriented and female-driven consumer culture in the 1980s," says Spielvogel.[7]

In other words, strong women, strong bodies. Psychologist Kathleen Pike, PhD, conducts research on women and body image in Japan. Her study "The Rise of Eating Disorders in Japan" explores the conflicting messages to which young Japanese women are exposed. On the one hand, the ideal of the homemaker and child-rearer is held aloft as the quintessential image of femininity—and is so strongly supported by the Japanese government that mothers who do not work outside the home receive subsidies. The transition from girlhood to womanhood, and from dependent child to self-sufficient adult, is marked by the transition into this domestic, maternal role.

On the other hand, Pike points out the "inherent contradictions" in a system that claims that the assumption of the role of homemaker and caretaker is a means of asserting independence. For young, professional Japanese women, what better way to make a statement about their resistance to "maturing" into this social role than to refuse the physical characteristics of a mother? "Whereas thinness in Western conceptualization is often associated with providing power and control, the Japanese pursuit of thinness is more reminiscent of a strategy for delaying maturation and the pursuant responsibilities," writes Pike.

Could it be that these body ideals aren't simply driven by the fear of becoming *a* mother, but a fear of becoming one's own mother? Every generation has its methods of marking a distinct cultural break with the previous one, from vocabulary to music. But surely the most obvious way to convey a generation's identity is through personal appearance. Nowhere is this use of the body as a symbolic break from the past more evident than in modern-day Japan. "The displacement of identity onto the body surface and concurrent increase in consumer products necessary for the attainment of these new body styles have overshadowed attributes formerly considered essential to the construction of female selves, particularly family status," notes Miller. In the last 15 years, a culture with rigid boundaries of gender behavior and a complex social hierarchy has witnessed radical changes in women's appearances and bodies—a shift that signals the social and political views of a new generation of Japanese women. Thin is still in, but breasts don't automatically have to mean maternity, and being more fit is clearly a sign of strength and autonomy.

Chihiro's Story

Women's ideas about beauty are created for themselves. They are in charge of their looks.

—CHIHIRO HAMANO, 30,
MAGAZINE WRITER, JIYUGAOKA

If you ask me, the body shape Japanese women are pursuing is a little scary. Young women are spending an incredible amount of time and money for beauty treatments at clinics and for memberships at gyms and health clubs. In my town alone, there are three new gyms and about five yoga studios.

There is a fairly precise idea that most Japanese women have for the ideal body: at least 5 feet 5 inches tall, around 110 pounds, and roughly 20 percent body fat. The ideal woman has a small face, small hips, long legs, long arms, and large chest—this, proportion-wise, is considered the best balance, and women with good-paying jobs are willing to go to great lengths to get it.

Since I was a preteen, "skinny is the best" is the mantra women follow. I do not fit the Japanese beauty ideal exactly. I am very, very short—about 4 feet 10 inches, but I am thin (I weigh just under 100 pounds). I have black, short, naturally curly hair (so I guess there, coincidentally, I fit the current craze for curls). I would never bleach or dye my hair, and I dislike the idea of getting a perm.

I was about 14 years old when I first started thinking about my appearance. It wasn't because of anything anyone said to me; it was just a gradual realization that I was very short. I became unhappy with my appearance because I had an inferiority complex about my height. There are many women like me in Japan, who are aware of the cultural ideal but know we will never meet it. When I was younger, I tried to be as charming as I could, to make up for in personality what I could not achieve in appearance.

As a woman, my thinking has changed. I am happy with my body. Now I think that everyone is beautiful when she or he is natural. I feel satisfied with my body and my face and my hair. This is who I am. Although I do go to the beauty salon about once a month, I am not part of the current gym and spa obsession sweeping Japan.

Sometimes there is a misunderstanding, that because Japanese women copy certain Western styles, that we also want to have a Western body. This is not exactly true. Yes, Japanese girls try to imitate a Western face, with pretty big eyes, whiter skin, blond or brown hair. But while our local TV shows may talk about "the latest method of body control of Madonna" or "the latest figure-shaping machines from the US," Japanese women do not want a glamorous, curvy body. They want a slim, trim body, but with more chest.

Women do not think about their bodies in terms of what men want. Japanese women want to be skinny because they are competitive with each other and because they love beautiful clothes and the newest fashions, and this is the body type that you can style most skillfully. They are willing to pay a lot of money to get it, too. I read in a magazine that young working women in Japan pay on average more than $300 every month for beauty procedures. Of course, many spend much more than that.

Calling the Shots

Having rejected the innocent baby-doll look and body of the 1980s, today's Japanese woman has a new body ideal: one that is lean, busty, and strong. She is fashionably dressed and can simultaneously take a business call while text-messaging her personal shopper on her way to the gym before a night out with the girls. In the United States, this is a look of conformity—of a woman trying to uphold the same standards as her peers, to be accepted, to fit a certain mold. In Japan, most anthropologists agree, this is the look of a woman breaking *free* from a mold, daring to be and look independent in a traditional society, and challenging her mother's notions of what a "mature" woman should look, act, and talk like. In adopting a new body ideal, this generation of financially independent women is signaling a break from the culture's past views of women.

"Women my age and younger are making more money than they ever have in our country," Kyoko Matsuda tells me. "And women see working on their appearance as an investment in themselves. For the same reason they like to buy nice clothes, they also love going to spas, getting treatments for their body, and trying new things that will make them look good. Japanese women hold themselves to a much higher standard of beauty than American women." What she means, she explains, is that Japanese women have traditionally always been thin.

So now, when they are investing in and "working on" their bodies, being thin and fit is taken to a whole new level. "It shows discipline," Kyoko explains. "What is a slim figure in the West is nowhere close to slim in the mind of a Japanese woman."

CHAPTER 10

AN AMERICAN IN PARADOX

"What size do you want to be?"
[the Caterpillar] asked.

"Oh, I'm not particular as to size,"
Alice hastily replied; "only one doesn't like
changing so often, you know."

The Caterpillar took the hookah out of its
mouth and yawned once or twice, and shook itself.
Then it got down off the mushroom, and crawled
away in the grass, merely remarking as it went,
"One side will make you grow taller, and the
other side will make you grow shorter."

—LEWIS CARROLL,
ALICE'S ADVENTURES IN WONDERLAND

"Now you really can have the perfect body you've always wanted, for less than you ever imagined. Come on, don't you want the best body your money can buy?"

Before I have the chance to roll over and hit the snooze button on my 6:00 a.m. alarm, I am greeted by this—a radio commercial for a new plastic surgery business, broadcast on the morning news. Our bodies, it seems, like cell phones, flat-screen televisions, and designer duds, are the latest objects worthy of an upgrade, and now is the time to get the new model at a bargain price.

Over the last decade in the United States, surgical procedures such as breast augmentation have increased by 142 percent, and non-surgical procedures such as Botox have skyrocketed by a whopping 743 percent. More than the latest designer jeans or must-have hand-bag, the perfect body tops every woman's wish list. It is her ultimate status symbol, a commodity she can work on, invest in, dress up, and pare down. And because it is uniquely hers, the body also serves as a blank slate upon which the American woman can etch her own story. As sociologist Debra Gimlin, PhD, notes,[1] we are living "in an era that has witnessed the decline of grand narratives of religion and politics that once provided meaning for people's lives. Because such changes have been accompanied by the increasing availability of technology for rationalizing the body, our physical being has come to be under-stood as one of the last arenas that we are able to control."

It's an important point, and one that helps explain, beyond media and marketing and gender pressures, why our culture is becoming increasingly obsessed with attaining the perfect body. Though our nation has historically prized individuality, we've always cherished certain moments of togetherness. Yet the last half-century has seen Americans become increasingly detached, self-oriented, and some-what indifferent to the shared mind-set that is inherent to many of our traditional cultural institutions. In 1950, more than half of the people in this country attended church; today, the number for regu-lar attendance is estimated to be below 20 percent. Community-based activities from neighborhood potlucks to Saturday night square dances are less frequently attended than they were 30 years ago. After-school team sports participation has also dropped. Even the family dinner table has far fewer people sitting around it these days—in a recent study, Americans reported 40 percent fewer meals shared with their families than they had in 1965. And though the current economic downshift may drive more people to make their own meals in an effort to save money, the fact that everyone in the family is eating at home doesn't necessarily mean that everyone in the family gathers around the dinner table for a shared meal. (Home-cooked meals are no guarantee that your kids won't still eat them while surfing the Internet, or that your husband will suddenly stop dining in front of the evening news.)

We are, increasingly, alone. We may still believe in God, but once we stop attending weekly religious services, the personal connection and obligation we feel to our religious communities rapidly diminishes. Of course we love our families, but regular visits to see the grandparents in their retirement home steal what precious free time we have, and phone calls to our siblings living in other states don't seem to fit into our hectic schedules. Our lives feel fully booked, even if they are empty of the type of social interactions that sustained previous generations. Instead, we live in an age of self-sufficiency and some might even say self-centeredness. As our identity becomes increasingly an inward-looking one, is it any wonder that we've chosen our bodies as the one thing we can control and use as the primary means of expressing who we are—or perhaps, who we want to be?

As economist Adam Smith outlined, it is human nature to strive toward the ultimate achievement, whether that's a six-figure salary or a size 2 silhouette. And the latter is, essentially, the ideal that is upheld by fashion icons, Hollywood, the media, and American women themselves. Tall, lanky, large breasted, small waisted. It is a figure that runs counter to the average—the last Centers for Disease Control figures show American women are 5 feet 4 inches and 165 pounds[2]—and an ideal well suited to our plentiful food culture (achieving such an ideal, after all, shows off the discipline required to just say no to the abundance of snacks and sweets that surround us each day).

So Why Aren't We Thinner?

Identifying the American ideal is the easy part. Trying to understand why we seem to be trending further and further away from our professed standard in our everyday lives is more complicated. We recognize that the body is a visual cue to a woman's social and economic status, and maintaining our appearance gives us an unquestionable edge over someone who does not. So why do we treat our bodies so poorly? Fueled by Coke, lattes, and value meals, sedated by alcohol, injected with Red Bull—for every artificial tool we use to keep our bodies functioning, there exists a healthier alternative. Sleep, exercise, vegetables, and fresh air are cheaper—but less immediately gratifying and more time consuming. We're short on time and patience these days, so instead, we cop to a culture that encourages pushing the limits of what our bodies can take, and when they show signs of protest, we look for the fast fix, purchasing expensive lotions, fad diets, and cosmetic procedures to set things right once again.

And as we've heard so much in the news lately, this body-punishing lifestyle is taking its toll on our health. Heart disease, diabetes, and obesity are on the rise. Stress-related disorders, from insomnia to anxiety, are up as well. The holistic medical community works hard to relay the message that long-term changes in lifestyle are necessary to reverse these disturbing trends. But for the most part, we don't seem to be taking their advice. We want an Rx that comes in a bottle or from a drive-thru window.

In our insta-world, it's only fitting in some ways that we pursue wellness—or "self-improvement"—with the same gusto for the fast, easy fix. Sure, we could eat healthfully, exercise, stay out of the sun . . . or we could have lipo. A tummy tuck. A microderm and a bit of Botox. A little time, a lot of money, but we can carry on with the lifestyle we enjoy. As Gimlin told me, "Again and again, the numerous women I've interviewed who had undergone plastic surgery rationalized their decision with the explanation that 'I am taking care of myself.' Meanwhile, the cost of such procedures is high, another indication of the economic status required for those who choose to undergo them. That leaves two groups of women who do not follow this route in pursuit of the perfect body: women who can't afford it, and women who prefer to commit themselves to a lifestyle of exercise and dieting to achieve the ideal body, and consider plastic surgery 'cheating.'" And of course, sometimes these groups are one and the same. Regardless of which camp they fall into, women who are actively pursuing a certain physical ideal will tell you they have made an "investment" in themselves to do so, whether it's a trip to their derm, a membership at Bally's, or a new pair of walking shoes.

But as our economic belts tighten, plastic surgeons, health clubs, and weight-management centers are also feeling the pinch. About 53 percent of plastic surgeons reported slower business in early 2008, according to a survey by the American Society for Aesthetic Plastic Surgery (ASAPS). It's not only cost that makes people hesitant to go under the knife, according to ASAPS findings, but the requisite time off from work. (Supporting this theory is the fact that Botox injections, one of the cheaper procedures with short recovery time, continued to grow in 2007, amounting to a $12.4 billion business.[3]) Gyms, too, have been affected by the economic downturn: Even those with monthly fees of $35 saw a drop in membership, from 42.7 million in 2006 to 41.5 million in 2007, according to the International Health, Racquet and Sportsclub Association.[4] (Although final 2008 figures are not yet available, a December 2008 survey by Opinion Research Corporation found that nearly one in five Americans is considering canceling gym memberships to save money.[5]) The United States is slowly becoming a nation where a woman's body shape can be used as an accurate determinant of whether or not she is recession-proof.

True, the contrast between the slims and the slim-nots is starker in tough economic times, but over the past 50 years we have gradually become a nation of extremes in the realm of appearance. At one end of the spectrum are the fashion models—5 feet 11 inches and 115 pounds, freaks of nature who happen to look fabulous in some of the most expensive clothes in the world. On the other end is the average American female, officially overweight at 165 pounds and 5 feet 4 inches. Clearly it is the first image we aspire to, which leads to this question: In America today, cars are bigger, beds are bigger, toilet seats are bigger, food portions are bigger, and homes are bigger. The only things getting smaller, it seems, besides cell phones and iPods, are the women we hold up as standards of physical perfection. Never before in our society has there been such a wide discrepancy between the average American body and the shape and size of our ideal. And the two ends of the spectrum seem to be growing further apart—the heavier we become, the smaller our models and actresses appear to shrink.

In a country with an overabundance of cheap, calorie-dense food, it's a challenge *not* to put on some extra pounds. It is perceived to be more expensive to eat "from nature"—meaning fruits and vegetables purchased in their whole form, which then need to be washed, peeled, chopped, and assembled—than it is to eat processed, prepared fast food. In a culture where 99-cent value meals abound, it is often believed that eating "skinny" means you've got money to burn.

But when we size up a woman's body shape, the assumptions we make go beyond her presumed income and move into the realm of her financial and personal priorities. Unlike the overweight person whom we often perceive to be sedentary, filling her evenings with television and junk food, our slim ideal leaves work and heads to the gym or to yoga class—or so we imagine. Afterward, she shops for organic produce, even if it costs 50 percent more. We perceive thin women as prioritizing their checkbooks to invest in themselves, whether or not they actually make big bucks. The slender girl is the one who budgets her money for Pilates classes and wholesome food. She is healthy, yes, and certainly, she looks good. But she is also somehow, in our minds, *better* than her heavier peers, and she is enviable. We aspire to look like her and to be like her.

Peter Stearns, PhD, a professor of history at George Mason University in Fairfax, Virginia, and author of *Fat History*, suggests that

America's obsession with thinness can be linked to a revolt against the overindulgence in which we've become mired, and the guilt that consumes us as we try to marry our Puritanical roots with our lust for material goods. "At its base, the need to fight fat remained a matter of demonstrating character and self-control in an age of excess," writes Stearns in his book, taking a look back at the evolution of our antifat stance in the last 50 years.[6] "Here surely was the reason that fat was long singled out over other known health problems. . . . Here was why fat was not fully a sickness in the ordinary sense. . . . Fat people should be able to control themselves. Even when doctors called fat women 'sick,' they meant morally or mentally defective, not uncontrollably ill. A decades-long history has produced firm convictions about appearance and physical fitness, to be sure, but undergirding both was a conviction that fat denoted bad character." Body size, Stearns suggests, can be altered by anyone with enough motivation—and it is for this reason that Americans tend to perceive slimness as not just a class indicator, but a means through which we communicate the values of piousness and self-control that are our cultural inheritance.

And just as the religiously devout feel guilty when they miss a day of worship or fail to abide by the tenets of their faith, so too does the person obsessed with becoming skinny feel guilty when her behavior runs contrary to her singular pursuit. Eat a muffin? Feel like a bad person. Guilt, it turns out, is a great motivator—feeling shameful about one's behavior is certainly an unpleasant emotional experience for which the natural reaction is to set matters straight. This works well, unless people discover a strategy of avoidance. Stearns believes this guilt-avoidance strategy reached new heights in the second half of the 20th century, not only when it came to our eating habits, but also other areas that made us feel uncomfortable. "The consumerist outlook in the 20th century was on the whole hostile to guilt, which was viewed as damaging," writes Stearns.[7] "Too much guilt, after all, called consumer indulgence into question; guilty people might feel they had to punish themselves by denying this purchase, that treat. The attack on fat, and particularly the ideal of battling weight through worried self-discipline, deliberately countered this overall discomfort with guilt."

Many Americans, however, increasingly rejected the notion that overeating was wrong. It seemed odd to deny oneself the jumbo soda or the oversize bagel when we were, at the same time, supersizing our houses and cars. Of course, in our current economic predicament, we now know that not all supersizing can be sustained; we've seen what happens when too many people put too many McMansions and SUVs on their credit cards without the means to pay them off. And as for those supersized meals, balancing the budget comes from calories burned equaling calories consumed, and consumption has definitely won the battle, leaving us with an obesity epidemic and a slew of health issues.

Pop Culture Cashes In

Given our preoccupation with body size and its connotations, perhaps it is not surprising that some of our most popular television shows involve, directly and indirectly, the evaluation of women's bodies. Of course, you could argue that virtually every woman on television, whether a news anchor or an actress, sports something pretty close to the ideal body. But I'm referring to programs like

America's Next Top Model and *The Biggest Loser,* where appearance is turned into a game with prizes for the winner.

America's Next Top Model is the second most popular show in its time slot for women ages 18 to 49: 1 million viewers tune in every week to watch a group of young beauties vie for a modeling contract.[8] The majority of the show's footage is comprised of fashion shoots and catwalk struts as the models attempt to impress a panel of judges. I can't help but wonder how the average, overweight American woman—the demographic for the show—derives any pleasure from watching this. And yet the devotion of its fans is astounding. *America's Next Top Model* offers an official online merchandise store and a message board with tens of thousands of postings, along with a chance to vote for your favorite model. What is it that the viewers find so appealing? Are they simply envious of those perfect bodies? Or (if you ask me, the more likely motive) is it entertaining, enjoyable, and on some level, reassuring, to see that even women who are model-worthy don't always get what they want? They cry, they confess their flaws, they get critiqued in humiliating detail by a panel of unforgiving industry experts. That, I think, is what keeps viewers coming back for more. It's comforting to know that even if we don't have an ideal body, those who do may not be as happy as we think they are.

The popularity of *The Biggest Loser* is in many ways easier to understand. We are a society of overweight people. The majority of these overweight people would prefer to be smaller. A 2007 survey by the International Food Information Council found that 70 percent of Americans in the past year had altered their diets in an attempt to lose weight. Moreover, 75 percent of respondents acknowledged being "concerned" about their weight, up 10 percent from only 1 year prior. And, in a separate study, 80 percent of fourth-grade girls admitted that they've tried to diet. Strangely, however, most Americans who admit to wanting to lose weight aren't terribly gung-ho about sticking with the plan. We all know the heavily cited statistic that 95 percent of diets fail, leading people to gain back the weight they lost—or more—within 5 years. And many of us don't even bother trying in the first place: In a 2008 NBC Universal/Meredith Corporation survey of 10,000 women across the United States, researchers found that weight loss was their number-one health concern; yet only one in two participants said they were willing to eat less and exercise regularly as a means of addressing their problem.

Watching the contestants on *The Biggest Loser* transform themselves from significantly obese to toned and trim—accomplishing what can feel impossible to those trying to lose weight at home—is inspiring, and it makes the show immediate and intimate to viewers' own battles of the bulge. Does it motivate them to take control of their own weight? Anecdotally, viewers say yes, the show provides a new incentive to stick with their diets.

As with *America's Next Top Model*, a number of profitable side businesses are affiliated with *The Biggest Loser*. The series airs in more than 90 countries; it has produced several *New York Times* best-selling books; and the show's now-famous trainers are featured in a handful of top-selling workout DVDs and books of their own. Despite media measurements that find a resistance to plus-size figures on television, could this be evidence that Americans do enjoy seeing people who look more like them on their favorite shows? Curious, and especially so in juxtaposition with shows like

America's Next Top Model, Project Runway, and *Dancing with the Stars,* where the participants are mainly svelte, Hollywood-attractive, and significantly out of reach (in body shape and in talent or lifestyle) for the average viewer. The secret to *The Biggest Loser*'s success, I think, is that its message (getting in shape is hard and requires focus and commitment, like an athletic competition) resonates with the viewer's own experience of how difficult it can be to lose weight and get in shape.

So as contestants on these shows whittle their way closer to our ideals—or angle for a glamorous modeling job because they already meet these ideals—the average viewer may be inclined to think that thin is not so unattainable after all. True, we might have to adjust a few inches here and there, and okay, there's no workout move that will magically take us from 5 feet 6 inches to 5 feet 10 inches, but through the massive pop culture lens of reality TV, we've seen that it's possible—if we really, *really* want to—to sculpt our bodies into a figure that loosely resembles the standard we've set for ourselves.

A Culture of Acceptance

For the vast majority of Americans, the numbers on the scale are moving only one way—and that's up. Our lifestyles are making it increasingly difficult for us to snag a piece of our fantasy body. "Over time, as people fail at their objective to be skinny, skinny becomes a useless motivational force," said a representative for Jenny Craig, speaking at the weight loss company's 2008 event to officially launch a new ad campaign. Their latest slogan: "Be your ideal size."

As I sat in a room for the launch luncheon with several dozen other New York magazine editors, it struck me that this tagline meant something very different to us than it does to the typical American woman. In New York City, and especially in our industry, the "ideal" by which many measure themselves can be found in the trim and fit models on our magazine's cover each month. But for the majority of Jenny Craig's target demographic, the proposition of working toward an "ideal size" theoretically takes the pressure off trying to be model-thin. The assumption is that the average American woman's ideal body would not, in fact, be a size 2, but would simply look like a better version of the body she already has—with a few extra pounds shaved off. Jenny Craig recognizes that the word *skinny* establishes a standard that feels unattainable, yet women still want to lose weight. So the company has essentially repackaged their weight loss message into language they hope is friendlier, less judgmental, less stressful. Because, as Jenny Craig's spokesperson points out, the pressure to be thin ceases to be an effective motivator if attempts at weight loss are consistently unsatisfactory in meeting that standard.

So perhaps what we really have are two ideals: the first, an iconic image of bodily perfection universally recognized on billboards and in magazines by the taut, lean look of air-brushed models; the second, a significantly modified version that feels much more plausible to the average woman. At *Fitness* magazine, the vast majority of readers who write to tell us their weight loss goals aspire to wear a dress size in the single digits again—a size 8, that is, not a size 2.

To aid these women on their way to achieving their "ideal size," Jenny Craig counsels on portion control and healthy-eating strategies. But their program (or any weight loss program, for that matter) cannot control one of the primary hindrances to our weight loss efforts: the instant access to food that has helped to pad the girth of the average American. No matter where you are, there is a snack supply within easy walking distance, and not the fresh fruit and vegetable snacks—minimal calories for maximum nutrients— but the processed, packaged, preserved stuff that nutritionists call empty calories. At the office? Try the vending machine. Out for a walk? There's always Starbucks. On the highway? Pull into the gas station for Cheetos, Fritos, or even a burger. We are inundated with food at every turn, and apparently, we haven't figured out how to just say no.

Food, for many, has become an addiction—we crave it even when we're not hungry; we think about it even when it's not mealtime. We hoard it (Two-4-One Special), we fear it (give away the kids' Halloween candy before I eat it!), we overindulge in it (all-you-can-eat buffet). But at the end of the day, food is not an addiction one can quit cold turkey, like cigarettes or alcohol. Food is something every body needs for survival; and unlike in countries with a food scarcity issue, where nature acts as a natural barrier to overconsumption, here in the United States, it's up to us to regulate the degree to which we take in calories. And that takes willpower and an ability to think long term—not just about our aesthetic ideals but about our health and the ramifications of instant gratification. The problem is, instant gratification is something Americans crave.

Our efforts to neutralize our love affair with fatty foods have become inspired more and more by breaking news from the medical community. The facts are eye-opening: Fat causes diabetes, heart disease, and increased cancer risk. But while every American hears about these problems on the evening news, the studies appear to have particularly strong impact on women of higher education levels, who also tend to be of higher socioeconomic status. In 2006, economists Mary Burke, at the Federal Reserve Bank of Boston, and Frank Heiland, in the department of economics at Florida State University in Tallahassee, published a study[9] in which they examined the various factors that make women with higher education more susceptible to messages about body size. The more educated a person, they hypothesized, the more likely it is that she reads the obesity statistics and understands the impact of weight on health; and most importantly, the more apt she is to be surrounded by a group of peers who are aware of the same information and apply pressure to each other to take action. In less-educated social circles, the flow of information about the health hazards of obesity isn't as strong; and at the same time, the social pressure among peers to lose weight is also less significant.

So the women armed with education and earning power indulge, then stress over their health; they overconsume, then swear to "be good." And not only is there peer pressure to be thin, but perhaps worse, there is also the self-imposed guilt based in the knowledge that they aren't treating their bodies as they know they should. Fatness is not just a size issue, but visible evidence that they are not properly caring for themselves. As Stearns says, "The image of fat as essentially evil, the result of personal failure . . . reinforced the link between prosaic diet literature and the need for a moral counterweight in a society of consumer indulgence."[10]

On the flip side, in the past 10 years America's Fat Pride movement has grown significantly. The number of women who have joined organizations like the National Association to Advance Fat Acceptance (NAAFA) is increasing—current membership stands at 11,000, with six national chapters. As NAAFA explains it, "Fat people are discriminated against in all aspects of daily life, from employment to education to access to public accommodations, and even access to adequate medical care. This discrimination occurs despite evidence that 95 to 98 percent of diets fail over 5 years and that 65 million Americans are labeled 'obese.' Our thin-obsessed society firmly believes that fat people are at fault for their size. . . . Fat discrimination is one of the last publicly accepted discriminatory practices. Fat people have rights and they need to be upheld!" The group's Web site, illustrated with the proud faces of fat Americans, also reports that weight discrimination in the workplace has doubled in the last decade, and that despite the fact that the majority of Americans are overweight, they are made to feel like the minority by a $49-billion-a-year diet industry.

But while it may be true that prejudice against overweight people persists, American society has also, in many ways, become increasingly supportive of the overweight person's lifestyle. Just look at the size of living room sofas, airplane seats, SUVs, toilets, and stretchy pants at the mall. Manufacturers have taken note of the ever-expanding waistlines of the American population and altered their products accordingly. You could argue that the fast-food chains that supersize meals are enabling the fat epidemic, but you could also argue that they are merely supporting what customers appear to want. We take no issue with Boeing, after all, or Jennifer Convertibles, when they offer seating options that would have dwarfed the average body half-a-century ago. Are they enabling an overweight lifestyle any more than are restaurants that cater to the consumer's desire for ever-bigger portions? Whose responsibility is it? For the member of a fat pride group, that answer is mutually satisfying to customer and business owner: It's nobody's responsibility, because there's nothing to be responsible for.

As we've seen evidenced throughout much of this book, in many economically challenged countries, larger female bodies are considered beautiful. So the question naturally arises: As the US economy sputters, will we witness the evolution of a similar cultural attitude? Stearns and others think we will, though that attitude might be born of different circumstances. In the 1980s, when levels of affluence began to recede, obesity began its rapid rise. During tough times, Americans see food as a viable indulgence, justifying their overconsumption—while still reporting that slimness is their ultimate goal—with the fact that food is one of their only remaining comforts, having had to scale back on other "luxury" items. "With no official relaxation of standards . . . Americans have become heavier," notes Stearns. "The pressure to seek solace and satisfaction in abundant food—another cultural tradition—has become ascendant."[11] On the other hand, the obesity boom that began in the '80s can also largely be traced to the growth of prepackaged, processed food, sold to consumers in larger and larger sizes. This time around, the recession had hit at a time when First Lady Michelle Obama was photographed planting a vegetable garden on the White House lawn. In many corners of our culture, fast food is falling out of favor. Whether that attitude will spread to the larger population remains to be seen.

No doubt about it, we are living in a paradox. As we pursue the

American version of perfection, the contradiction between what we say we want and how we choose to live doesn't seem to show any signs of being reconciled. Where once skin color, religion, and nationality were used as an artificial means of separating people into different classes, we have ironically reinstated the policies of division with a new set of superficial social rules.

CHAPTER 11

THE BODY OF TOMORROW

There is one thing, though, that has not and can never
be commoditized—and that is imagination.

—THOMAS FRIEDMAN, *THE WORLD IS FLAT*

In 2008, one of our country's most popular forms of sporting entertainment—watched by seven to nine million American fans every week—announced that big changes were afoot for the upcoming season. NASCAR unveiled a new racing car—one with an increased number of standardized parts to level the playing field and prevent owners from buying their way into the winner's circle. Far from its Southern, blue-collar, stock car racing roots, 21st-century NASCAR had evolved into a sport in which the team that could afford the better engine, chassis, or suspension was predictably the team who won—not necessarily the team with the best driver. With a new set of standards for the racing car, NASCAR promised fans they would experience a better, more exciting competition. The focus of the event would return to the talent of the drivers, not which team had more money.

They called it the Car of Tomorrow.

Whether or not the Car of Tomorrow has been a success depends on whom you ask. Drivers grumble that it does not handle as well as its previous incarnation; fans complain that it is uniformly slower on the track—and what is car racing about, if not speed? But the one thing everyone does seem to agree on is that now the real heroes on any given Sunday at the track are the drivers with the greatest skill, discipline, and finesse behind the wheel. One supposes that the drivers who work the hardest to maximize their cars' potential will reap the biggest rewards.

Over in the distant world of beauty, a similar revolution and revelation is beginning to unfold. Today's ideal body is on the verge of being traded in for a new model. Like NASCAR's leveled playing field, equal access to a slim figure in America is becoming a very real possibility.

There are already signs that over-the-counter skinny is coming: At the GlaxoSmithKline research laboratories, scientists have developed the so-called antifat pill, Alli, which enables the body to block up to 25 percent of the fat a person consumes and is the only Food and Drug Administration–approved over-the-counter weight loss supplement. (The underlying drug, orlistat, is also sold by prescription as Xenical.) At St. Vincent's Institute in Melbourne, Australia, chemists are exploring a pill that mimics the effect of exercise to increase weight loss. The institute's director, Tom Kay, says the pill synthetically reproduces the naturally occurring protein inside our cells that works as a "fuel gauge" during exercise to regulate how food is turned into usable energy for the body. Other pharmaceutical companies are investigating a pill that would prevent the body from absorbing extra calories after its daily limit is met. And beyond the pharmaceutical counter, anyone who spends a few hours in the bookstore will encounter rows of paperbacks that detail what to eat, how much, and when, to reach a goal weight. Some are bunk, but many are backed by basic science: 3,500 calories equals 1 pound; to shed 1 pound in 1 week, you need to consume 500 fewer calories per day. Need help with the tricky math? Online calorie trackers and even iPhone apps will do it for you.

Of course, unlike a pill, a diet plan—however easy—does require motivation and discipline. But either way, in the not-too-distant future, skinny—once the hallmark of supermodels and socialites— will be easier to attain for everyday Janes. So what happens when the look of the elite can be bought at the local drugstore? If thin becomes mass-market accessible, will our body ideal be as "ideal" as it once was? Where would be the allure in a shape so available, so pedestrian? In fact, one wonders if part of the reason we're still striving for skinny is that we simply haven't come up with a better model. It's a fair question, I think: In lieu of the pursuit of thin, what body shape would women chase?

It doesn't seem likely that the pendulum will swing back to the full, fleshy figures that were popular centuries ago. Most Americans already have that body, and we're more aware than ever of the health-related hazards that come with being overweight, as well as the financial burden that accompanies the pounds. In fact, a recent Medicare study has found that the average nonoverweight woman costs the medical system $6,224 a year, while an obese woman costs $9,612—or 33 percent more.[1]

A recent report in the *Journal of Physical Activity and Health*[2] estimates the total national costs of physical inactivity at $251 billion annually, and the cost for excess weight at $257 billion. (The estimates included healthcare costs, workers' compensation, and productivity loss.) As it currently stands, 66 percent of Americans are overweight, and today's generation of children is the first in our history to be at risk for lower life expectancy than their parents, due to weight-related diseases. Add to this the troubling news that the rising cost of health insurance means that 75 million Americans are rolling the dice and going without, and you can piece together the makings of an economic health tsunami.

The Rise of Skinny-Fat

At a 2008 press conference in New York City, I had the opportunity to talk with Barbara Rolls, PhD, creator of the Volumetrics eating plan. I asked her what she thought American women might look like 15 years down the road.

"More of the same, unfortunately," she said. "I don't see Americans making any drastic changes in their approach to food. It is too ingrained in us, this idea of more is better. If it's left up to the consumer, I do not think you are going to see a widespread sea change in how we eat. If there is going to be change, it's going to happen because the scientists found a way to intervene by artificially lessening the calorie content of the foods we love."

Rolls's theory that there will be an increase in the manufacture and availability of reduced-calorie foods has already hit supermarket shelves: lite ice cream, fat-free cheese, baked potato chips—lower-calorie versions of our favorite foods abound. But what Rolls suggests goes even further: Soon we'll be able to shop for "light" pasta, low-cal rice, maybe even reduced-calorie potatoes.

But will it matter? We've been cutting calories via "diet foods" for nearly 3 decades now, and Americans have only been getting fatter. Either our bodies just aren't fooled by the fake stuff we substitute for the higher caloric items or—probably more likely—the psychology of calorie-reduced foods backfires. Rather than reducing the amount people are eating, lower-cal food substitutes have actually increased overall consumption by enabling the consumer to rationalize: "Since this is good for me, I can eat more of it."

Whether it's a magic pill, a diet book, or a redesigned potato, it seems likely that science will play a role in the ideal body of tomorrow. And while science increasingly tells us that obesity can cause cardiovascular disease, it also tells us that getting skinny does not grant immunity from it. In fact, even skinny is starting to get a bad rap. A study in the December 5, 2007, issue of the *Journal of the American Medical Association* found that people with higher fitness levels, regardless of body size, lived longer than their thinner but less-fit peers.[3] Study coauthor Steven Blair, MD, a former president of the American College of Sports Medicine and a longtime proponent of exercise as a treatment for health issues, reports that individual fitness levels are a better indicator of health than a person's weight and proposes that fitness tests should be used as a measurement of a patient's wellness during annual checkups.

It's a lot for the American woman to digest: Fat is unattractive, fat is bad for your health, skinny is sexy—no, skinny is bad for your health, too? It feels like a frustrating double standard. Adding to the debate, a hybrid of both of these body types has earned its own pop culture terminology: skinny-fat. This recently coined term is defined (in one of five possible definitions) by the online source www. urbandictionary.com as "[a] term used when a person is thin, yet does not eat healthy or take care of themselves. . . ." "Skinny-fat" is used to describe Hollywood starlets who seem to survive on little more than cigarettes and black coffee, and who may be able to wear a size 2 but who probably can't run 2 miles. Skinny-fat bodies may be small, but they earn the second half of their label because what little there is of them is so lacking in muscle strength and definition, they might as well be overweight couch potatoes.

So where does that leave us? Being thin is no longer enough—the Body of Tomorrow will have to be more special and more difficult to attain in order to be granted "ideal" status. And like NASCAR's Car of Tomorrow, which was constructed to showcase the skill and effort of individual drivers, I suspect that our new body ideal will be a similar reflection of an individual's hard work. We will move from a society that rewards skinniness as an achievement in its own right to one that recognizes fitness as the evidence of dedication and skill.

Danielle's Story

Everyone wants the quick fix. But more women are finding huge satisfaction in making a long-term commitment to their body, too.

—DANIELLE BLOOM, 38, SINGER, NASHVILLE

I can't pinpoint one thing that started my issues with my body, but I do remember a moment that added to my already growing insecurity. I was dating this guy in high school, and I really liked him. I wanted to do something nice, so I went out and bought a card for him. The card said, "Thank you for never saying those three little words: You look fat." (It was high school, what can I say!) But before I gave it to him, we started talking and sure enough, the topic of body size came up. I almost died when he said to me, "Yeah, you're a little chunky; you could stand to lose a few pounds." I didn't become anorexic because of that, but it didn't help.

I moved to Nashville to pursue a career in music when I was 19. Before then, I saw the skinny models in advertisements or these perfect-looking women on TV, but it didn't bother me so much. It was when I started getting involved in the entertainment business and I began looking for other singers to model myself after that I started questioning my body even more. I'd look at someone and say, "I need to look like her to get signed." I cut way back on what I was eating and started working out like crazy. In my mind, I just wasn't pretty enough, thin enough. All women are insecure on some level, but in the music world, sex sells. It can be hard to get away from the obsession with how you look.

I started fainting a lot, waking up in the middle of the night to heart palpitations. At the time, I didn't connect the fact that I was getting too thin with my health problems. Finally, I called my mom, and she sent me straight to see a doctor. It took a while, but I got better. I think American women want a quick fix. We want to wake up in the morning and think, "Wow, I've got the body of my dreams." We don't want to have to work for it, and a fit body is something you have to work at.

After recovering from my eating disorder, I had this epiphany about taking better care of my body. I committed myself to living a healthy lifestyle. I am getting my personal trainer certification so I can show women how to get the body they want in a healthy way. There is so much satisfaction in going to the gym, working hard on your body, and seeing results in sculpted muscles and having more energy. Yes, it takes work. But it gives me confidence in how I look in a way that unhealthy dieting never could.

Fit Is the New It

I recently had coffee with a friend who was remodeling her kitchen. She brought along several brochures for the new cabinet doors she was considering. Each of the choices was a nicely crafted white door with inlaid panels and silver knobs. I studied the three identical-looking photos and asked her: "What's the difference?"

"About $15,000," she said. "One is solid maple, one is plywood, and one is Thermofoil—not even real wood!"

By appearance alone, I would have been happy with any of them. But later that afternoon, we stopped by the store where the cabinets were on display. I opened and closed each one, feeling the weight of the doors give and resist as they moved. The Thermofoil,

I realized, was like a piece of plastic—light, unsteady, and unsub-
stantial. The solid maple door, meanwhile, meant business, sound-
ing a satisfying "thud" as it closed against its wooden frame. It was
clearly the higher-end choice—not immediately apparent from a
photograph, but obvious once you actually felt the material and put
the door to use.

These days, we can buy knockoff accessories on the cheap (just
take a trip to New York City's Chinatown if you need a bargain "Louis
Vuitton" handbag), and reproductions of everything from shoes to
watches have become incredibly convincing imitations. But there is
always a market for the *real* deal—constructed with time, care, and
from the highest-quality materials.

Which means . . . hello, Gabrielle Reece; so long, Paris Hilton.
The body ideal of tomorrow will require that a woman is slim with
substance. I think it's safe to say that the new prerequisites for an
ideal body will include a hearty devotion to exercise and body sculpting. Not in a bodybuilder sort of way, mind you, but in a "look at my
yoga-toned arms" fashion that reveals in one quick flash—or flex—
that you are a woman of determination, ambition, discipline, and
success. You are the "real deal."

Already the trend is starting to emerge, led in part by the very
admirably toned figure of First Lady Michelle Obama, whose seem-
ing body confidence, not to mention buff biceps, has set a new bar
for accomplished women everywhere. Even before the era of
Michelle's sleeveless ensembles, a 2006 study conducted by the Centers for Disease Control and Prevention found a 25 percent increase
over the past 10 years in the number of women who incorporate
weights into their workouts. Researchers attribute this trend to a

wider appreciation of a fit body shape, as well as heightened awareness among women of the importance of strength training as an
integral part of osteoporosis-preventing bone health (the greatest
increase was found in the 65-plus category, with a 66 percent jump
in regular weight lifters).[4]

As always, money is never far from the ideal body equation.
High-end, designer gyms and expensive workouts with celebrity
trainers are already en vogue. The more sculpted and toned a woman's body, the more time one assumes the woman has been able to
devote to her pursuit of physical perfection. And time—today as it
was yesterday—is a valuable commodity. The more you have to
spare on leisurely pursuits, the thinking goes, the richer you must
be. But *having* time and choosing to spend it on strenuous activity
are two different matters, just as the ability to purchase the fanciest cardio equipment and hire brand-name personal trainers
doesn't guarantee a woman will work out. That's a key difference
between thin and fit—thin requires the discipline *not* to do something (eat), while fit requires an additional exertion of yourself,
which many would say makes it even more of a challenge. And so
the ante for the ideal body in America has just been upped a
notch—layered on top of the economic factors that contribute to it
and thereby allow our bodies to serve as status symbols, there is a
new psychological variable. She with the fittest body is not only
a financial success, she is disciplined, motivated, and mentally
strong: the elite of the elite.

The fit body is one of a woman's own making. It requires an investment of one of our most limited resources: time. It's the resource most
often cited for thwarting our best fitness intentions: According to an

American Heart Association survey, 69 percent of American women set a goal to work out more in 2007, but only 22 percent succeeded due to time constraints.[5] And it's not just a matter of committing in short spurts. Sexy muscle definition doesn't happen overnight; six-pack abs and killer V-shaped calves are the culmination of months of daily workouts—not the 30-minutes-on-the-treadmill type, but the painstakingly deliberate, focused, sweat-laden sort. The Body of Tomorrow belongs to the woman who wakes up at 5:00 a.m. to hit the gym, then comes home and feeds the kids, drops them at school, and powers her way through her high-pressure day at the office. In this way, our fantasy figure may approach the body and mind ideals of Japan—I believe that we will increasingly view our buff bodies as a reflection of our internal qualities: tough, ambitious, and motivated. Research is beginning to bear this out as well. A national survey of female executives at the top of their corporation's food chain revealed that four out of five played competitive sports growing up and two-thirds still worked out regularly and included strength training in their routines (a number that is double the national average). We perceive women with strong bodies to be successful, and statistically it turns out they *are* some of the highest-paid and most powerful women in America.

The strong-body ideal offers another reward for women, aside from a great physique: the empowering knowledge of what their bodies can *do*. This, I think, is another reason the fit look will catch on. It is personally satisfying to cross the finish line of your first 5-K; it is also yet another measure by which you can size yourself up to others. And unlike body shape, which is changeable only within certain genetic limitations, for the recreational athlete, the potential for fitness improvement is vast, and satisfaction from the incremental increases in strength and speed and muscle tone provides regular feedback and incentive to stick with it.

Another trend has emerged that gives credence to the rise of fit as ideal: the recent spike in female participation in endurance sporting events, from marathons to triathlons. Road Runners Club of America, reports a fairly steady membership since the mid-1980s, though one of the organization's largest chapters, New York Road Runners, notes that this membership swell reflects a decline in male participants and a 15 percent increase in female runners.[6] Women's sports apparel maker Danskin, meanwhile, has seen participation in its triathlons grow from 150 participants in 1990 to well over 5,000.[7] Overall, female membership for USA Triathlon, a tri-enthusiast national organization, has tripled in the past 15 years. The introduction of charity-based training groups has aided in the attraction for a female audience. One of the biggest national organizations, the Leukemia Society's Team in Training, reports that 75 percent of their members are women. In all cases, the trend is toward a young, affluent demographic—under 40 years old and likely to be earning more than $80,000 a year.[8]

Don't get me wrong: Participants in these endurance sports still represent a minute portion of the American female demographic. But upward spikes in participation do suggest that the bar is being raised on tomorrow's ideal—one where looking the part will no longer be a free pass, and the proof will be in the bench press.

Fitness industry experts say that the shift is already under way: A February 2008 survey of health club facilities nationwide by IDEA Health & Fitness Association found that one in three gyms reported the use of traditional cardio equipment such as stairclimb-ers was in decline, while 40 percent said the use of dumbbells and other free weights was increasing.[9] Does this mean we're heading toward an era of Dara Torres–inspired physiques? Kathie Davis, executive director of IDEA, says, "More than ever, we live in a cul-ture that takes its cues from celebrities. And right now, it's very 'in' for celebrities to want to look toned. Our studies suggest they are doing at least equal parts cardio and strength training in their workouts, which is vastly different than the old days when the emphasis was on dieting."

When IDEA started out in 1982, the fitness industry was in its infancy. No one had a personal trainer, Davis points out, unless they were trying to get in shape for a movie role. High-impact aerobics was the extent of our fitness wisdom for women. From its inception as a $3 million business back then to its astronomical expansion into a $15 billion enterprise today,[10] the secret to the fitness industry's success has been its ability to sell women a sense of control over their "flaws," which are constantly highlighted by the beauty industry. Beauty marketing has always been about buying a product that will "fix" you. Fitness marketing focuses on "fixing" yourself.

Such a can-do sales pitch is clearly resonating with American women, who increasingly say they work out to build themselves up mentally and physically, rather than simply to lose weight. Hence a 72 percent increase in gyms offering grueling, military-inspired "boot camp" classes.[11] "We've gone from Jane Fonda in a mirrored studio to outdoor boot camps that mimic army training," Davis tells me. "The trend is definitely towards fit, not thin. Fifteen years from now, I would imagine this distinction will only grow greater, as members of the fitness industry innovate new ways to push and test your body. *Being strong* will be the real badge to wear."

And this, it strikes me, is putting our imaginations to use for a happily positive, proactive future: a society in which women aspire to be slim and strong, and one that has moved beyond that quaint time in our past where simply being skinny was good enough to call yourself a success.

CONCLUSION

*If the stars should appear but one night every
thousand years how man would marvel and stare.*

—RALPH WALDO EMERSON

*There is a vitality, a life force, an energy, a
quickening, that is translated through you into
action, and because there is only one of you in all
time, this expression is unique.*

—MARTHA GRAHAM

In this book I have presented research and examples of bodies
around the globe with the goal of shining a light on the unique
cultural and historical context that has helped to shape and per-
petuate foreign (and domestic) body ideals. I realize it might seem
as though I believe the physical aesthetics of a culture are somehow
immune to the influences of globalization—I don't. Fiji and the
South Pacific islands are not alone in their rapid conversion to an
appearance standard that was once opposite to their native values.
The women of the countries I chose to feature exemplify, to me,
some of the most diverse and interesting aesthetic values that can
be found—values from which American women could learn a lot.
Many of us could gain needed perspective from the South African

perception that a beautiful body is one that reflects good health, or the Jamaican belief that the body is an expression of the rhythms of its people. In the global exchange of body ideals, I hope that such attitudes can find a way of merging into our own beliefs.

Appearance versus Attitude

I chose not to dedicate space in this book to examining the body attitudes of some of the world's most highly acclaimed bodies—such as those of French and Italian women—but I do think it is worth mentioning that while the physical manifestations of, say, American and French ideals are alike in many ways, the efforts put forth to achieve such body types tend to be remarkably different. The French, renowned as a culture for their sophistication and elegance, seem to approach the care and feeding of their bodies with the same attitude of refinement: They eat delicious, fresh foods, consumed in moderation. Are there exceptions? Of course. The golden arches and other food franchises have permeated virtually every corner of the world, and Paris is no exception. But by and large, food in France—and many other European countries—is a metaphor for life. It is meant to be savored and celebrated, not abused, exceedingly measured, or painfully restricted.

It's a stark contrast to the approach taken by many American women who practice self-restraint with great gusto, only to gorge later on the very foods they've sworn off. But despite the difference in attitude of how we go about attaining the perfect body, in the end, the actual body ideals for European and American women are more alike than not. In fact, though French women might not profess to aspire to the super-skinny shape of Hollywood starlets, they come closer to achieving this body type than do their American counter-parts. A 2009 study from France's National Institute of Demographic Studies found that while France has the highest percent of underweight women of any European country at just over 6 percent, only half of them consider themselves to be thin, suggesting that the French body ideal is actually smaller than that of other European countries and America.

The thin woman denotes different qualities of character in different countries, but ultimately, the larger connotation is the same. In Europe, thinness is typically indicative of a woman who enjoys her life and takes care of herself properly. In America, such thinness is a sign of education, willpower, and discipline, along with economic advantage. In both cases, it is symbolic of a woman who has achieved her society's definition of success, and the perception of status and class that accompanies it.

Worth Your Weight in Gold?

What does it say about human values if at the end of the day our physical ideals can be boiled down to dollars and cents? These days, affluence is suspect—the bubble of our economy has burst, people are losing their homes and being denied credit, our jobs are in jeopardy, and the high rollers who had a hand in getting us into this mess—and profited from it—are regarded with disdain. Wealth has come to be associated with extravagance and irresponsibility. In these economically troubled times, when thrift and caution have become fashionable, will we still want to emulate the look of the elite?

The answer, I think, is yes. So far, at least, our body ideal seems to be holding steadier than our currency. Now more than ever, we value the qualities conveyed by the ideal body: that hard work, discipline, ambition, and willpower can make a difference—that good old-fashioned elbow grease can help us meet our goals. Qualities that in better times have yielded financial success are now valued for their potential to help us ride out the uncertainty of today's markets. Our bodies are vehicles to convey this sentiment: We are strong and determined; we will persevere.

END NOTES

Introduction

1. J. H. Crowther, E. M. Wolf, and N. Sherwood, "Epidemiology of Bulimia Nervosa," in *The Etiology of Bulimia Nervosa: The Individual and Familial Context,* ed. M. Crowther, D. L. Tennenbaum, S. E. Hobfoll, and M. A. P. Stephens (Washington, DC: Taylor and Francis, 1992), 1–26.

Also: C. G. Fairburn, P. J. Hay, and S. L. Welch, "Binge Eating and Bulimia Nervosa: Distribution and Determinants," in *Binge Eating: Nature, Assessment, and Treatment,* ed. C. G. Fairburn and G. T. Wilson (New York: Guilford, 1993), 123–43.

Also: H. W. Hoek, "The Distribution of Eating Disorders," in *Eating Disorders and Obesity: A Comprehensive Handbook,* ed. K. D. Brownell and C. G. Fairburn (New York: Guilford, 1995), 207–11.

Also: H. W. Hoek and D. van Hoeken, "Review of the Prevalence and Incidence of Eating Disorders," *International Journal of Eating Disorders* 34, no. 4 (2003): 383–96.

Also: C. M. Shisslak, M. Crago, and L. S. Estes, "The Spectrum of Eating Disturbances," *International Journal of Eating Disorders* 18, no. 3 (1995): 209–19.

2. Statistics from National Eating Disorders Association.

3. A. Case and A. Menendez, "Sex Differences in Obesity Rates in Poor Countries: Evidence from South Africa," *National Bureau of Economics Research Working Paper* no. 13541, p. 24–25, (2007).

4. N. Wolf, *The Beauty Myth: How Images of Beauty Are Used against Women* (New York: Harper Perennial, 1990), 13.

Chapter 1

1. D. Buss, "Sex Differences in Human Mate Preferences: Evolutionary Hypotheses Tested in 37 Cultures," *Behavioral and Brain Sciences* 12, no. 1 (1989): 1–49.

2. F. Marlowe and A. Wetsman, "Preferred Waist-to-Hip Ratio and Ecology," *Personality and Individual Differences* 30, no. 3 (2001): 481–89.

Also: F. W. Marlowe, C. L. Apicella, and D. Reed, "Men's Preferences for Women's Profile Waist-Hip-Ratio in Two Societies," *Evolution and Human Behavior* 26 (2005): 458–68.

3. G. Rhodes and T. Tremewan, "Averageness, Exaggeration, and Facial Attractiveness," *Psychological Science* 7 (1996): 105–10.

4. D. Symons, *The Evolution of Human Sexuality* (New York: Oxford, 1981), 195–96.

5. N. Etcoff, *Survival of the Prettiest* (New York: Random House, 1999), 145.

6. American Academy of Facial Plastic and Reconstructive Surgeons Annual Survey, 1993, Washington, DC, as cited in N. Etcoff, *Survival of the Prettiest* (New York: Random House, 1999), 146.

7. T. Judge and D. Cable, "The Effect of Physical Height on Workplace Success and Income: Preliminary Test of a Theoretical Model," *Journal of Applied Psychology* 89, no. 3 (2004): 428–41.

8. R. Thornhill and S. Gangestad, "Human Facial Beauty," *Human Nature* 4, no. 3 (1993): 237–69.

Also: K. Grammer and R. Thornhill, "Human (*Homo Sapiens*) Facial Attractiveness and Sexual Selection: The Role of Symmetry and Averageness," *Journal of Comparative Psychology* 108, no. 3 (1994): 233–42.

Also: C. A. Samuels, G. Butterworth, T. Roberts, L. Graupner, and G. Hole, "Facial Aesthetics: Babies Prefer Attractiveness to Symmetry," *Perception* 23 (1994): 823–31.

9. M. Livio, *The Golden Ratio: The Story of Phi, The World's Most Astonishing Number* (New York: Broadway, 2003).

Also: B. Atalay, *Math and the Mona Lisa: The Art and Science of Leonardo da Vinci* (Washington, DC: Smithsonian Books, 2004).

10. www.beautyanalysis.com

11. "Women CEOs for Fortune 500 Companies," *Fortune*, April 17, 2006.

Chapter 2

1. A. Smith, *The Wealth of Nations*, Book Two, Chapter III (1776).

2. G. Boeree, *Personality Theories* (1997), copyright George Boeree (e-textbook).

3. GM cars sold in second quarter 2007, 2.4 million: *Dow Jones Newswire*, July 2007. Sales of Ferrari 2008 total worldwide, 6,400: *The Weekly Driver*, January 2008.

4. L. Spielvogel, *Working Out in Japan: Shaping the Female Body in Tokyo Fitness Clubs* (Durham, NC: Duke University Press, 2003).

Also: M. Featherstone, "The Body in Consumer Culture," in *The Body: Social Process and Cultural Theory*, M. Featherstone, M. Hepworth, and B. Turner, eds., (London: Sage Press, 1991), 170–96.

5. D. Gimlin, *Body Work: Beauty and Self-Image in American Culture* (Berkeley and Los Angeles: University of California Press, 2002), 14.

6. D. Gimlin, *Body Work: Beauty and Self-Image in American Culture* (Berkeley and Los Angeles: University of California Press, 2002), 2.

Chapter 3

1. S. Goldhill, *Love, Sex & Tragedy: How the Ancient World Shapes Our Lives* (Chicago: University of Chicago Press, 2004), 11–28.

2. K. Clark, *The Nude: A Study in Ideal Form* (Princeton, NJ: Princeton University Press, 1956, 1972, 1984, 1990), 13.

3. K. Clark, *The Nude: A Study in Ideal Form* (Princeton, NJ: Princeton University Press, 1956, 1972, 1984, 1990), 356.

4. V. Swami, K. Poulogianni, and A. Furnham, "The Influence of Resource Availability on Preferences for Human Body Weight and Non-human Objects," *Journal of Articles in Support of the Null Hypothesis*, 4 (2006): 17–28.

Also: V. Swami and A. Furnham, *The Psychology of Physical Attraction* (London: Routledge, 2008).

5. P. Howden-Chapman and J. Mackenbach, "Poverty and Painting: Representations in 19th Century Europe," *British Medical Journal* 325 (2002):1502–05.

6. "Prevalence of Overweight and Obesity Among Adults: United States 2003–2004," a report from the Centers for Disease Control and Prevention's National Center for Health Statistics (NCHS), 2006.

Also see: C. L. Ogden, M. D. Carroll, L. R. Curtin, M. A. McDowell, C. J. Tabak and K. M. Flegal. "Prevalence of Overweight and Obesity in the United States, 1999–2004," *Journal of the American Medical Association* 295 (2006): 1549–55.

Chapter 4

1. S. Brownell, interview with author for *Marie Claire* magazine, "Women's Bodies: Then and Now," April 2004.

2. "China Rises to World's Eighth Largest Beauty Market," *China Economic Review*, November 7, 2003.

Also: J. Hellstrom, "Estee Lauder to Beat Market Growth in China," *Reuters*, December 11, 2006.

3. *Merrill Lynch/CapGemini 2007 World Wealth Report.*

4. A. Haworth, "Nothing about These Women Is Real," *Marie Claire*, July 2005: 64.

5. Fabrice Aghassian, head of research and development for L'Oreal Paris, interview with author.

Chapter 5

1. M. Steinberg and S. Johnson, "Hitting Home: How Households Cope with the HIV/AIDS Epidemic," report for Henry J. Kaiser Foundation and Health Systems Trust (October 2002).

2. M. Faber and H. S. Kruger, "Dietary Intake, Perceptions Regarding Body Weight, and Attitudes toward Weight Control of Normal Weight, Overweight, and Obese Black Females in a Rural Village in South Africa," *Ethnicity and Disease* 15, no. 2 (2005): 238–45.

3. T. Puoane, J. M. Fourie, M. Shapiro, L. Rosling, N. C. Tsaka, A. Oelofse, "Big Is Beautiful—An Exploration with Urban Black Community Health Workers in a South African Township," *South African Journal of Clinical Nutrition* 18, no. 1 (2005): 6–15.

4. D. Yach and A. S. Marks, "Complex and Controversial Causes for the 'Obesity' Epidemic," *International Journal of Medical Marketing* 4, no. 3 (2004): 288.

5. S. Dubner, "Why Are Women More Likely to Be Obese Than Men?" *New York Times*, October 26, 2007.

6. J. Seed, paper on South African women and eating disorders presented at British Psychological Society, April 16, 2004.

7. S. Day, "Natural Hairstyles Assert Identity in Post-Apartheid South Africa," *South Africa in Transition: News, Feature, and Comment* (March 1999), UC Berkeley School of Journalism.

Chapter 6

1. E. Sobo, *The Sweetness of Fat: Health, Procreation and Sociability in Rural Jamaica* (New York: Routledge, 1997): 256–71.

2. E. Sobo, *The Sweetness of Fat: Health, Procreation and Sociability in Rural Jamaica* (New York: Routledge, 1997): 256–71.

3. S. Harter, "Causes and Consequences of Low Self-Esteem in Children and Adolescents," in *Self-Esteem: The Puzzle of Low Self-Regard*, ed. R. F. Baumeister (New York: Plenum, 1993).

Also: S. Harter, *The Construction of Self: A Developmental Perspective* (New York: Guilford Press, 1999).

4. E. Anderson-Fye, "A Coca-Cola Shape: Cultural Change, Body Image, and Eating Disorders in San Andres, Belize," *Culture, Medicine and Psychiatry* 28 (2004): 561–95.

5. P. Cramer and G. Anderson, "Ethnic/Racial Attitudes and Self-Identification of Black Jamaican and White New England Children," *Journal of Cross-Cultural Psychology* 34 (2003): 395–416.

Chapter 7

1. P. Rantanen, "Non-Documentary Burqa Pictures on the Internet: Ambivalence and the Politics of Representation," *International Journal of Cultural Studies* 8, no. 3 (2005): 329–51.

Chapter 8

1. A. E. Becker, *Body, Self, and Society* (Philadelphia: University of Pennsylvania Press, 1995), 38.

2. A. E. Becker, *Body, Self, and Society* (Philadelphia: University of Pennsylvania Press, 1995), 50.

3. E. J. Strahan, A. E. Wilson, K. E. Cressman, and V. M. Buote, "Comparing to Perfection: How Cultural Norms for Appearance Affect Social Comparisons and Self-Image," *Body Image* 3, no. 3 (2006): 211–27.

Also: D. Trampe, D.A. Diederik, and F. W. Siero, "On Models and Vases: Body Dissatisfaction and Proneness to Social Comparison Effect," *Journal of Personality and Social Psychology* 92, no. 1 (2007): 106–18.

4. E. J. Strahan, S. J. Spencer, and M. P. Zanna, "Don't Take Another Bite: How Sociocultural Norms for Appearance Affect Women's Eating Behavior," *Body Image* 4, no. 4 (2007): 331–42.

5. L. McLaren, "Socioeconomic Status and Obesity," *Epidemiologic Reviews* 29 (2007): 29–48.

6. "Weekly Newsletter Update," *South Pacific Tourism Organization*, issue no. 159 (2007).

7. "Regional Tourism Body Eyes $2 Billion by 2010," *Fiji Times*, February 17, 2007.

8. "Travel and Tourism Economic Impact Annual Report," *World Travel and Tourism Council*, March 1, 2009.

9. L. K. Williams, L. A. Ricciardelli, M. P. McCabe, G. G. Waqa, and K. Bavadra, "Body Image Attitudes among Indigenous Fijian and European Australian Adolescent Girls," *Body Image* 3 (2006): 275–87.

Chapter 9

1. L. Miller, *Beauty Up: Exploring Contemporary Japanese Body Aesthetics* (Berkeley and Los Angeles: University of California Press, 2006), 78.

2. "Bokura no Raifusutairu Hakusho," *Fine Boys* magazine, no. 142 (1998): 183–90.

3. T. Screech, *Sex and the Floating World* (Honolulu: University of Hawaii Press, 1999): 100.

4. Author interview with Takie Libra.

5. L. Miller, *Beauty Up: Exploring Contemporary Japanese Body Aesthetics* (Berkeley and Los Angeles: University of California Press, 2006), 78.

6. P. Constantine, *Japanese Slang Uncensored* (Tokyo: Yenbooks, 1994).

7. L. Spielvogel, *Working Out in Japan: Shaping the Female Body in Tokyo Fitness Clubs* (Durham, NC: Duke University Press, 2003), 31.

Chapter 10

1. D. Gimlin, "The Absent Body Project: Cosmetic Surgery as a Response to Bodily Dys-Appearance," *Sociology* 40, no. 4 (2006): 699–716.

2. "Mean Body Weight, Height, and Body Mass Index (BMI) 1960–2002: United States," a *National Health and Nutrition Examination Survey*, conducted by the Centers for Disease Control and Prevention's National Center for Health Statistics (NCHS), 2004.

3. "2007 National Average for Physician/Surgeon Fees Per Procedure," *The American Society for Aesthetic Plastic Surgery* (2007).

4. "2008 IHRSA Global Report: The State of the Health Club Industry," annual report from the International Health, Racquet, and Sportsclub Association (IHRSA), 2008.

5. "Fitness and Finances" survey, conducted by Opinion Research Corporation, December 2008.

6. P. Stearns, *Fat History: Bodies and Beauty in the Modern West*, 2nd ed. (New York: NYU Press, 2002), 117.

7. P. Stearns, *Fat History: Bodies and Beauty in the Modern West*, 2nd ed. (New York: NYU Press, 2002), 147.

8. "'Model' Struts through Tough Time Slot," *The San Diego Union-Tribune*, March 2, 2007.

9. M. Burke and F. Heiland, "The Strength of Social Interactions and Obesity among Women," in *Agent-Based Computational Modelling*, ed. F. Billari, T. Fent, A. Prskawetz, and J. Scheffran (Heidelberg, Germany: Physica Verlag, 2006).

Also: M. Burke and F. Heiland, "Social Dynamics of Obesity," *Economic Inquiry* 45, no. 3 (July 2007): 571–91.

10. P. Stearns, *Fat History: Bodies and Beauty in the Modern West*, 2nd ed. (New York: NYU Press, 2002), 256.

11. P. Stearns, *Fat History: Bodies and Beauty in the Modern West*, 2nd ed. (New York: NYU Press, 2002), 256.

Chapter 11

1. M. L. Daviglus, K. Liu, L. L. Yan, A. Pirzada, L. Manheim, W. Manning, D. B. Garside, R. Wang, A. R. Dyer, P. Greenland, and J. Stamler, "Relation of Body Mass Index in Young Adulthood and Middle Age to Medicare Expenditures in Older Age," *Journal of the American Medical Association* 292, no. 22 (2004): 2743–49.

2. D. Chenoweth and J. Leutzinger, "The Economic Cost of Physical Inactivity and Excess Weight in American Adults," *Journal of Physical Activity and Health* 3, no. 2 (2006).

3. X. Sui, M. J. LaMonte, J. N. Laditka, J. W. Hardin, N. Chase, S. P. Hooker, and S. N. Blair, "Cardiorespiratory Fitness and Adiposity as Mortality Predictors in Older Adults," *Journal of the American Medical Association* 298, no. 21 (2007): 2507–16.

4. J. Kruger, S. Carlson, H. Kohl III, "Trends in Strength Training—United States, 1998–2004," *Morbidity and Mortality Weekly Report*, Division of Nutrition and Physical Activity, National Center for Chronic Disease Prevention and Health Promotion, Centers for Disease Control and Prevention, 55, no. 28 (July 21, 2006): 769–72.

5. "Choose to Move 2007," national survey by the American Heart Association (September 2007).

6. Foxnews.com interview with Becky Lambros, executive directive of Road Runners Club of America, July 5, 2005.

7. Danskin Women's Triathlon Series.

8. "Female Runner Profile," National Runner Survey, Running USA Organization, 2007.

9. *IDEA Fitness Programs and Equipment Survey*, IDEA Health and Fitness Association, July 2008.

10. Author interview with Kathie Davis, executive director, IDEA.

11. *IDEA Fitness Programs and Equipment Survey*, IDEA Health and Fitness Association, July 2008.

INDEX

Boldface page references indicate photographs.

M

Male dominance theory, 11–14
Miss Plastic Surgery pageant, 60–61,
  60
Money. *See also* Economics
  in ancient Greece, 31–32
  body ideal steadier than,
    192–93
  body size and, 76
  Coca-Cola-bottle shape and, 90
  cosmetics costs in China, 55
  cosmetic surgery and, 52,
    59–60
  Fijian body size and, 131
  fitness tied to, 185
  height correlated with, 7
  influence on art, 37–38
  needed for ideal body, 20–21
  poverty, 38–40, 46, 49, 112
  slimness tied to, in US, 164
  South African body size and, 70

N

Neck, emphasized in Japan, 147
Nudes in art, 25–26, 28–32, 35–37

O

Obesity. *See also* Curves
  costs of, 178–79
  in Fiji, 132
  socioeconomic development and,
    137–38
  in South Africa, 70, 76, 77
  in US, 174
Orlistat antifat drug, 177

P

Pale skin in China, 51–52, 57
People's Republic. *See* China
Perseus Liberating Andromeda,
  37
Pharmaceutical aids, 177–78

Phi (golden ratio), 9–11, 28, **29**
Plastic surgery. *See* Cosmetic
  surgery
Poverty. *See also* Money
  in Afghanistan, 112
  in Communist China, 46,
    49
  post-Industrial, 38–40
Prejudice against fat in US, 43–44,
  164, 165, 173, 175
*Proportions of the Human Figure,
  The,* **29**
Prototypicality theory, 7–9

S

Schoolgirl look in Japan, 151
Self-actualization, 16–17
Self-esteem, 22, 24
Self-improvement, 15–16, 160–61
Skinny-fat, 180–81, 182–83
Slimness. *See also* Eating disorders;
  Weight loss
  in Afghanistan, 111, 112, 117
  in Communist China, 46, 49,
    63
  in Europe vs. US, 191–92
  in Fiji, 131, 134
  fitness vs., 180–81, 184–89
  in Jamaica, 90–91, 99
  in Japan, 153–54, 156, 157
  pharmaceuticals aiding,
    177–78
  post-Industrial, 38–39
  skinny-fat, 180–81, 182–83
  in socially oriented art, 40
  in South Africa, 69, 70–71,
    72–73
  TV promoting, 134, 136–37, 138
  US attitudes, 164, 165–66
  as youthfulness, 23
South Africa. *See also* South African
  black women
  "big is beautiful" ideal, 69, 73,
    75–76, 77–78
  HIV/AIDS in, 67–69, 70–73